D0901524

THE CHRONIC DISEASES

THEIR PECULIAR NATURE AND THEIR HOMOEOPATHIC CURE

By

DR. SAMUEL HAHNEMANN

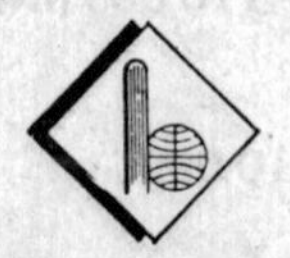

B. JAIN PUBLISHERS PVT. LTD.
NEW DELHI - 110 055

Price : Rs. 25.00

Reprint Edition : 1993
© Copyright with the Publisher
Published by :
B. Jain Publishers Pvt. Ltd.
1921, Street No. 10, Chuna Mandi
Paharganj, New Delhi - 110 055 (INDIA)
Printed at :
J. J. Offset Printers
Kishan Kunj, Delhi - 110 092

ISBN 81—7021—016—X

BOOK CODE B-2265

CONTENTS.

PUBLISHERS' PREFACE.

This volume, which contains the theoretical part of Hahnemann's CHRONIC DISEASES, has been issued at the urgent request of several Professors in Homœopathic Medical Colleges, who wish to use it as a college text book. It is to be hoped, too, that the profession at large will appreciate this volume, which in the opinion of many ranks in importance with the ORGANON.

INTRODUCTION

Messers B. Jain Publishers have approached me for giving my views regarding the publication of the theoretical part of the Chronic Diseases written by Dr. Samuel Hahnemann. From my student days this small but valuable book has served me as guide like Organon. In this book the life experience of Dr. Samuel Hahnemann has been incorporated. It throws a light on the burning zeal in the heart of our Master for the allereation of Human Suffering. During his long experience and careful case recording, he noticed that there was something due to which patients treated on the basis of Similimum got recurrence of the same troubles after some time. This set him thinking that there was something lacking in the fundamental laws laid down in the Organon, due to which permanent cure was not taking place. The underlying cause could not escape his acute observation and careful persual of the recorded cases. He came to the conclusion that the hindrance in the permanent cure of chronic cases was due to Chronic Miasms present in the affected persons. This let to the foundation of the theory of Chronic Diseases which is his last gift to the profession and the suffering humanity.

I have always stressed the need for a careful and intelligent study of this most valuable book to my students. It has served me as a guideline all through my practice and has given me chances of effecting remarkable cures in cases of chronic ailments. The conception of Psora and the list of symptoms of Latent Psora given by Hahnemann are really marvellous things and serve as a guide to the student as well as the busy practitioner in different cases. Every time one gives a reading to this book he will discover new gems in it. The Organon and the Theory of Chronic Diseases are two books which reveal new thoughts and inspiration every time one gives a reading to them as Gita opens a new door to the divine light every time one gives a reading to it. The practical approach in the treatment of Psora, Syphilis and Sycosis given in he book really serves as a guideline in the treatment of all types of chronic ailments. I strongly recommend it to the students to give a thorough and careful reading to this book and they will never fail in the treatment of chronic causes if they follow carefully the instructions given in the book.

Shanti Dev

(SHANTI DEV)
B.Sc., D.M.S., M.H.M.S.,
M.A.S.F., Vaidya Shiromani
Physician Incharge, Central
Government Health Scheme.
Homoeopathic Dispensery,
New Delhi

New Delhi.
Dated : 24th May, 1972

AUTHOR'S PREFACE

TO THE FIRST EDITION—1828

If I did not know for what purpose I was put here on earth—to become better myself as far as possible and to make better everything around me that is within my power to improve—I should have to consider myself as lacking very much in worldly prudence to make known for the common good, even before my death, an art which I alone possess, and which it is within my power to make as profitable as possible by simply keeping it secret.

But in communicating to the world this great discovery I am sorry that I must doubt whether my contemporaries will comprehend the logical sequence of these teachings of mine, and will follow them carefully and gain thereby the infinite benefits for suffering humanity which must inevitably spring from a faithful and accurate observance of the same, or whether, frightened away by the unheard of nature of many of these disclosures, they will not rather leave them untried and uninitiated and, therefore, useless.

At least I cannot hope that these important communications will fare better than the general Homoeopathy, which I have published hitherto. From unbelief in the efficacy of the small and attenuated doses of medicine, which I made known to the medical world after a thousand warning trials, as being the most efficient (distrusting my faithful asseverations and reasons), men prefer to endanger their patients for years longer with large and larger doses. Owing to this, they generally do not live to see the curative effects, even as was the case with myself before I attained this diminution of dose. The cause of this was that it was overlooked that these doses by their attenuation were all the more suitable for their homoeopathic use owing to the development of their dynamic power of operation.

What would men have risked if they had at once followed my directions in the beginning, and had made use of just these small doses from the first? Could anything worse have happened than that these doses might have proved inefficient? They surely could do no harm! But in their injudicious, self-willed application of large doses for homoeopathic use they only, in fact *only* once again, went over that roundabout road so dangerous to their patients in order to reach the truth, which I myself had already successfully passed over, and indeed with trembling, so as to save them this trouble; and if they really desired to heal, they were nevertheless at last compelled to arrive at the only true goal, after having inflicted many an injury and wasted a good part of their fair life. All this I had already laid before them faithfully and frankly, and had long before given them the reasons.

May they do better with the great discovery herewith presented to them! And if they should not treat this discovery any better—well, then a more conscientious and intelligent posterity will alone have the advantage to be obtained by a faithful, punctual observance of the teachings here laid down, of being able to deliver mankind from the numberless torments which have rested upon the poor sick owing to the numberless, tedious diseases, even as far back as history extends. This great boon had not been put within their reach by what Homoeopathy had taught hitherto.

PREFACE TO THE FOURTH VOLUME.*

INQUIRY INTO THE PROCESS OF HOMŒOPATHIC HEALING.

We have no means of reaching with our senses or of gaining essential knowledge as to the process of life in the interior of man, and it is only at times granted us to draw speculative conclusions from what is happening as to the manner in which it may have occurred or taken place; but we are unable to furnish conclusive proofs of our explanations from the changes which are observed in the organic kingdom; for the changes in living organic subjects have nothing in common with those taking place in what is organic, since they take place by processes entirely different.

It is, therefore, quite natural that in presenting the Homœopathic Therapeutics I did not venture to explain how the cure of diseases is effected by operating on the patient with substances possessing the power to excite very similar morbid symptoms in healthy persons. I furnished, indeed, a conjecture about it, but I did not desire to call it an explanation, *i. e.*, a definite explanation of the modus operandi. Nor was this at

*The work on the "Chronic Diseases" was originally published in five parts, and every part, except the second, had its own preface, discussing some questions of general interest to Homœopathy.—*Transl.*

all necessary, for it is only incumbent upon us to cure similar symptoms correctly and successfully, according to a law of nature which is being constantly confirmed; but not to boast with abstract explanations, while we leave the patients uncured, for that is all which so-called physicians have accomplished.

These physicians have made many objections to the explanation I have given, and they would have preferred to reject the whole homœopathic method of curing (the only one possible) merely because they were not satisfied with my efforts at explaining the mode of procedure which takes place in the interiors of man during a homœopathic cure.

I write the present lines, not in order to satisfy those critics, but in order that I may present to myself and to my successors, the genuine practical Homœopaths, another and more probable attempt of this kind toward an explanation. This I present because the human mind feels within it the irresistible, harmless and praiseworthy impulse to give some account to itself as to the mode in which man accomplishes good by his actions.

As I have elsewhere shown, it is undeniable that our vital force, without the assistance of active remedies of human art, cannot overcome even the slight acute diseases (if it does not succumb to them) and restore some sort of health without sacrificing a part (often a large part) of the fluid and the solid parts of the organism through a so-called crisis. How our vital force effects this, will ever remain unknown to us; but so much is sure, that this force cannot overcome even these diseases in a direct manner, nor without such sacrifices. The Chronic Diseases, which spring from miasms, cannot be healed unaided, even by such sacrifices, nor can real health be restored by this force alone. But it is just as certain that even if this force is enabled by the true (homœopathic) healing art, guided by the human understanding, to overpower and overcome (to cure) not only the quickly transient, but also the chronic diseases arising from miasms in a direct manner and without such sacrifices, without loss of body and life, nevertheless, it is always this power, the vital force, which conquers. It is in this case as with the army of a country, which drives the enemy out of the country; this army ought to be called victorious, although it may not have won the victory without foreign auxiliaries. It is the organic vital force of our body which cures natural diseases of every kind directly and without any sacrifices as soon as it is enabled by means of the correct (homœopathic) remedies to win the victory. This force would not, indeed, have been able to conquer without this assistance, for our organic vital force, taken alone, is only sufficient to maintain the unimpeded progress of life so long as man is not morbidly affected by the hostile operation of forces causing disease.

Unassisted, the vital force is no match to these hostile powers; it hardly opposes a force equal to the hostile operation, and this, indeed, with many signs of its own sufferings (which we call morbid symptoms). By its own power our vital force would never be able to overcome the foe of chronic disease, nor even to conquer transient diseases, without considerable losses inflicted on some parts of the organism, if it remained without external aid, without the assistance of genuine remedies. To give such support is the duty enjoined on the physician's understanding by the Preserver of life.

As I have said above, our vital force *hardly* opposes *an equal* opposition to the foe causing the disease, and yet no enemy can be overcome except by a superior force. Only homœopathic medicine can give this superior power to the invalidated vital force.

Of itself this vital principle, being only an organic vital force intended to preserve an undisturbed health, opposes only a weak resistance to the invading morbific enemy; as the disease grows and increases it opposes a greater resistance, but, at best, it is only an equal resistance; with weakly patients it is not even equal, but weaker. This force is neither capable, nor destined, nor created for an overpowering resistance, which will do no harm to itself.

But if we physicians are able to present and oppose to this instinctive vital force its morbific enemy, as it were magnified through the action of homœopathic medicines—even if it should be enlarged every time only by a little—if in this way the image of the morbific foe be magnified to the apprehension of the vital principle through homœopathic medicines, which, in a delusive manner, simulate the original disease, we gradually cause and compel this instinctive vital force to increase its energies by degrees, and to increase them more and more, and at last to such a degree that it becomes far more powerful than the original disease. The consequence of this is, that the vital force again becomes sovereign in its domain, can again hold and direct the reins of sanitary progress, while the apparent increase of the disease caused by homœopathic medicines disappears of itself as soon as we, seeing the preponderance of the restored vital force, *i. e.*, of the restored health, cease to use these remedies.

The fund or the fundamental essence of this spiritual vital principle, imparted to us men by the infinitely merciful Creator, is incredibly great, if we physicians understand how to maintain its integrity in the days of health, by directing men to a healthy mode of living, and how to invoke and augment it in diseases by purely homœopathic treatment.

PREFACE TO FIFTH VOLUME.

DILUTIONS AND POTENCIES (DYNAMIZATIONS).

Dilutions, properly so-called, exist almost solely in objects of taste and of color. A solution of salty and bitter substances becomes continually more deprived of its taste the more water is added, and eventually it has hardly any taste, no matter how much it may be shaken. So, also, a solution of coloring matter, by the admixture of more and more water, becomes at last almost colorless, and any amount of shaking will not increase its color.

These are, and continue to be, real attenuations or dilutions, but no dynamizations.

Homœopathic Dynamizations are processes by which the medicinal properties, which are latent in natural substances while in their crude state, become aroused, and then become enabled to act in an almost spiritual manner on our life; *i. e.*, on our sensible and irritable fibre. This development of the properties of crude natural substances (dynamization) takes place, as I have before taught, in the case of dry substances by means of trituration in a mortar, but in the case of fluid substances, by means of shaking or succussion, which is also a trituration. These preparations cannot be simply designated as dilutions, although every preparation of this kind, in order that it may be raised to a higher potency, *i. e.*, in order that the medicinal properties still latent within it may be yet farther awakened and developed, must first undergo a further attenuation, in order that the trituration or succussion may enter still further into the very essence of the medicinal substance, and may thus also liberate and expose the more subtle part of the medicinal powers that lie hidden more deeply, which could not be effected by any amount of trituration and succussion of the substances in their concentrated form.

We frequently read in homœopathic books that, in the case of one or another person in a certain case of disease, some high (dilution) dynamization of a medicine was of no use at all, but a lower potency proved effectual, while others have seen more success from higher potencies. But no one in such cases investigates the cause of the great difference of these effects. What prevents the preparer of the medicines (and this ought to be the homœopathic physician himself; he himself ought to forge and whet the arms with which to fight the disease)--what prevents him, in preparing a potency, from giving 10, 20, 50 and more succussive strokes against a somewhat hard, elastic body to every vial containing one drop of the lower potency with 99 drops of alcohol, so as to obtain strong potencies? This would be vastly more effective than giving only a few nerveless succussive strokes, which will produce little more than dilutions, which ought not to be the case.

The perfection of our unique art of healing and the welfare of the patients seem to make it worth while for the physician to take the trouble necessary to secure the utmost efficiency in his medicines.

Modern wiseacres have even sneered at the 30th potency, and would only use the lower, less developed and more massive preparations in larger doses, whereby they have been, however, unable to effect all that our art can accomplish. If, however, every potency is dynamized with the same number of succussive strokes, we obtain, even in the fiftieth potency, medicines of the most penetrating efficacy, so that every minute pellet moistened with it. after being dissolved in a quantity of water, can and must be taken in small parts, if we do not wish to produce too violent an action with sensitive patients, while we must remember that such a preparation contains almost all the properties latent in the drug now fully developed, and these can only then come into full activity.

PARIS, December 19th, 1838.

Nature of Chronic Diseases.

The Homœopathic healing art, as taught in my own writings and in those of my pupils, when faithfully followed, has hitherto shown its natural superiority over any allopathic treatment in a very decided and striking manner; and this not only in those diseases which suddenly attack men (the acute diseases), but also in epidemic diseases and in sporadic fevers.

Venereal diseases also have been radically healed by Homœopathy much more surely, with less trouble and without any sequelæ; for without disturbing or destroying the local manifestation it heals the internal fundamental disease from within only, through the best specific remedy. But the number of the other chronic diseases on this great earth has been immeasurably greater, and remains so.

Treatment by allopathic physicians hitherto merely served to increase the distress from this kind of disease; for this treatment consisted of a whole multitude of nauseous mixtures (compounded by the druggist from violently acting medicines in large doses, of whose separate true effects they were ignorant), together with the use of manifold baths, the sudorific and salivating remedies, the pain-killing narcotics, the injections, fomentations, fumigations, the blistering plasters, the exutories and fontanels, but especially the everlasting laxatives, leeches, cuppings and starving treatments, or whatever names may be given to all these medicinal torments, which continually varied like the fashions. By these means the disease was either aggravated and the vital force, spite of so-called tonics used at intervals, was more and more diminished; or, if any striking change was produced by them, instead of the former sufferings, there appeared a worse state—nameless diseases caused by medicine, far worse and more incurable than the original natural one—while the physician consoled the patient with the words: "The former sickness I have been fortunate enough to remove; it is a great pity that a new (?) disease has appeared, but I hope to be as successful in removing this latter as in the former." And so, while *the same disease assumed various forms*, and while new diseases were being added by the use of improper, injurious medicines, the sufferings of the patient were continually aggravated until his pitiable lamentations were hushed forever with his dying breath, and the relatives were soothed with the comforting pretense: "Everything imaginable had been used and applied in the case of the deceased."

It is not so with Homœopathy, the great gift of God!

Even in these other kinds of chronic diseases, its disciples, by following the teachings presented in my former writings and my former oral lectures, accomplished far more than all the afore-mentioned methods of curing, *i. e.*, when they found the patient not too much run down and spoiled by allopathic treatment, as was unfortunately too often the case where the patient had any money to spend.

Using the more natural treatment, Homœopathic physicians have frequently been able in a short time to remove the chronic disease which they had before them, after examining it according to all the symptoms perceptible to the senses; and the means of cure were the most suitable among the Homœopathic remedies, used in their smallest doses which had been so far proved as to their pure, true effects. And all this was done without robbing the patient of his fluids and strength, as is done by the allopathy of the common physicians; so that the patient, fully healed, could again enjoy gladsome days. These cures indeed have far excelled all that allopathists had ever—in rare cases—been able to effect by a lucky grab into their medicine chests.

The complaints yielded for the most part to very small doses of that remedy which had proved its ability to produce the same series of morbid symptoms in the healthy body; and, if the disease was not altogether too inveterate and had not been too much and in too great a degree mismanaged by allopathy, it often yielded for a considerable time, so that mankind had good reason to deem itself fortunate even for that much help, and, indeed, it often proclaimed its thankfulness. A patient thus treated might and often did consider himself in pretty good health, when he fairly judged of his present improved state and compared it with his far more painful condition before Homœopathy had afforded him its help.*

* Of this kind were the cures of diseases caused by a psora not yet fully developed, which had been treated by my followers with remedies which did not belong to the number of those which,

Even some gross errors of diet, taking cold, the appearance of weather especially rough, wet and cold or stormy, or even the approach of autumn, if ever so mild, but, more yet, winter and a wintry spring, and then some violent exertion of the body or mind, but particularly some shock to the health caused by some severe external injury, or a very sad event that bowed down the soul, repeated fright, great grief, sorrow and continuous vexation, often caused in a weakened body the re-appearance of one or more of the ailments which seemed to have been already overcome; and this new condition was often aggravated by some quite new concomitants, which if not more threatening than the former ones which had been removed homœopathically were often just as troublesome and now more obstinate. This would be especially the case whenever the seemingly cured disease had for its foundation a psora which had been more fully developed. When such a relapse would take place the Homœopathic physician would give the remedy most fitting among the medicines then known, as if directed

---

later, proved to be the chief anti-psora remedies; because these remedies were not yet known. They had been merely treated with such medicines as Homœopathically best covered and temporarily removed the then apparent moderate symptoms, thus causing a kind of a cure which brought back the manifest psora into a latent condition and thus produced a kind of healthy condition, especially with young, vigorous persons, such as would appear as real health to every observer who did not examine accurately; and this state often lasted for many years. But with chronic diseases caused by a psora already fully developed, the medicines which were then known never sufficed for a complete cure, any more than these same medicines suffice at the present time.

against a new disease, and this would again be attended by pretty good success, which for the time would again bring the patient into a better state. In the former case, however, in which merely the troubles which seemed to have been removed were renewed, the remedy which had been serviceable the first time would prove less useful, and when repeated again it would help still less. Then perhaps, even under the operation of the Homœopathic remedy which seemed best adapted, and even where the mode of living had been quite correct, new symptoms of disease would be added which could be removed only inadequately and imperfectly; yea, these new symptoms were at times not at all improved, especially when some of the obstacles above mentioned hindered the recovery.

Some joyous occurrence, or an external condition of circumstances improved by fortune, a pleasant journey, a favorable season or a dry, uniform temperature, might occasionally produce a remarkable pause of shorter or longer duration in the disease of the patient, during which the Homœopath might consider him as fairly recovered; and the patient himself, if he good-naturedly overlooked some passable moderate ailments, might consider himself as healthy. Still such a favorable pause would never be of long duration, and the return and repeated returns of the complaints in the end left even the best selected Homœopathic remedies then known, and given in the most appropriate doses, the less effective the oftener they were repeated. They served at last hardly even as weak palliatives. But usually, after repeated attempts to conquer the disease which appeared in a form always somewhat changed, residual complaints appeared which the Homœopathic medicines hitherto proved, though not few, had to leave uneradicated, yea, often undiminished. Thus there ever followed varying complaints ever more troublesome, and as time proceeded, more threatening, and this even while the mode of living was correct and with a punctual observance of directions. The chronic disease could, despite all efforts, be but little delayed in its progress by the Homœopathic physician and grew worse from year to year.

This was, and remained, the quicker or slower process in such treatments in all non-venereal, severe chronic diseases, even when these were treated in exact accordance with the Homœopathic art as hitherto known. Their beginning was promising, the continuation less favorable, the outcome hopeless.

Nevertheless this teaching was founded upon the steadfast pillar of truth and will evermore be so. The attestation of its excellence, yea, of its infallibility (so far as this can be predicted of human affairs), it has laid before the eyes of the world through facts.

Homœopathy *alone* taught *first of all* how to heal the well-defined idiopathic diseases, the old, smooth scarlet fever of Sydenham, the more recent purples, whooping cough, croup, sycosis, and autumnal dysenteries, by means of the specifically aiding Homœopathic remedies. Even acute pleurisy, and typhous contagious epidemics must now allow themselves to be speedily turned into health by a few small doses of rightly-selected Homœopathic medicine.

Whence then this less favorable, this unfavorable, result of the continued treatment of the non-venereal chronic diseases even by Homœopathy? What was the reason of the thousands of unsuccessful endeavors to heal the other diseases of a chronic nature so that lasting health might result? Might this be caused, perhaps, by the still too small number of Homœopathic remedial means that have so far been proved as to their pure action? The followers of Homœopathy have hitherto thus consoled themselves; but this excuse, or so-called consolation, never satisfied the founder of Homœopathy—particularly because even the new additions of proved valuable medicines, increasing from year to year, have not advanced the healing of chronic (non-venereal) diseases by a single step, while acute diseases (unless these, at their commencement, threaten unavoidable death) are not only passably removed, by means of a correct application of Homœopathic remedies, but with the assistance of the never-resting, preservative vital force in our organism, find a speedy and complete cure.

Why, then, cannot this vital force, efficiently affected through Homœopathic medicine, produce any true and lasting recovery in these chronic maladies even with the aid of the Homœopathic remedies which best cover their present symptoms; while this same force which is created for the restoration of our organism is nevertheless so indefatigably and successfully active in completing the recovery even in severe acute diseases? What is there to prevent this?

The answer to this question, which is so natural, inevitably led me to the discovery of the nature of these chronic diseases.

To find out then the reason why all the medicines known to Homœopathy failed to bring a real cure in the above-mentioned diseases, and to gain an insight more nearly correct and, if possible, quite correct, into the true nature of the thousands of chronic diseases which still remain uncured, despite the incontestable truth of the Homœopathic Law of Cure, this very serious task has occupied me since the years 1816 and 1817, night and day; and behold! the Giver of all good things permitted me within this space of time to gradually solve this sublime problem through unremitting thought, indefatigable inquiry, faithful observation and the most accurate experiments made for the welfare of humanity.*

It was a continually repeated fact that the non-venereal chronic diseases, after being time and again removed Homœopathically by the remedies fully proved up to the present time, always returned in a more or less varied form and with new symptoms, or reappeared annually with an increase of complaints. This

* Yet I did not allow any of these unintermitted endeavors to become known either to the world or to my followers, not, indeed, because the ingratitude so frequently shown to me prevented me, for I heed neither ingratitude nor persecutions on my troublous path of life, which yet has not proved altogether joyless, because of the great goal toward which I have striven. No, I left it unmentioned because it is improper, yea, hurtful to speak or write of things still immature. Not until the year 1827 did I communicate the essentials of the discovery to two of my pupils, who had been of the greatest service to the art of Homœopathy, for their own benefit and that of their patients, so that the whole discovery might not be lost to the world if perchance a higher call to eternity had called me away before the completion of the book—an event not so very improbable in my seventy-third year.

fact gave me the first clew that the Homœopathic physician with such a chronic (non-venereal) case, yea, in all cases of (non-venereal) chronic disease, has not only to combat the disease presented before his eyes, and must not view and treat it as if it were a well-defined disease, to be speedily and permanently destroyed and healed by ordinary Homœopathic remedies, but that he has always to encounter only some separate fragment of a more deep-seated original disease.

The great extent of this disease is shown in the new symptoms appearing from time to time; so that the Homœopathic physician must not hope to permanently heal the separate manifestations of this kind in the presumption, hitherto entertained, that they are well-defined, separately existing diseases which can be healed permanently and completely. *He, therefore, must first find out as far as possible the whole extent of all the accidents and symptoms belonging to the unknown primitive malady* before he can hope to discover one or more medicines which may Homœopathically cover the whole of the original disease by means of its peculiar symptoms. By this method he may then be able victoriously to heal and wipe out the malady in its whole extent, consequently also its separate members; that is, all the fragments of a disease appearing in so many various forms.

But that the original malady sought for must be also of a *miasmatic*, chronic nature clearly appeared to me from this circumstance, that after it has once advanced and developed to a certain degree it can never be removed by the strength of any robust constitution, it can never be overcome by the most wholesome diet and order of life, nor will it die out of itself. But it is evermore aggravated, from year to year, through a transition into other and more serious symptoms,* even till the end of man's life, like every other chronic, miasmatic sickness, *e. g.*, the venereal bubo which has not been healed from within by mercury, its specific remedy, but has passed over into venereal disease. This latter, also, never passes away of itself, but, even with the most correct mode of life and with the most robust bodily constitution, increases every year and unfolds evermore into new and worse symptoms, and this, also, to the end of man's life.

I had come thus far in my investigations and observations with such non-venereal patients, when I discovered, even in the beginning, that the obstacle to the cure of many cases which seemed delusively like specific, well-defined diseases, and yet could not be cured in a Homœopathic manner with the then proved medicines, seemed very often to lie in a former eruption of itch, which was not unfrequently confessed; and the beginning of all the subsequent sufferings usually dated from that time. So also with similar chronic patients who did not confess such an infection, or, what was probably more frequent, who had, from

---

* Not unfrequently phthisis passes over into insanity; dried-up ulcers into dropsy or apoplexy; intermittent fever into asthma; affections of the abdomen into pains in the joints or paralysis; pains in the limbs into hemorrhage, etc. and it was not difficult to discover that the later diseases must also have their foundation in the original malady and can only be a part of a far greater whole.

inattention, not perceived it, or, at least, could not remember it. After a careful inquiry it usually turned out that little traces of it (small pustules of itch, herpes, etc.) had showed themselves with them from time to time, even if but rarely, as an indubitable sign of a former infection of this kind.

These circumstances, in connection with the fact that innumerable observations of physicians,* and not infrequently my own experience, had shown that an eruption of itch suppressed by faulty practice or one which had disappeared from the skin through other means was evidently followed, in persons otherwise healthy, by the same or similar symptoms; these circumstances, I repeat, could leave no doubt in my mind as to the internal foe which I had to combat in my medical treatment of such cases.

Gradually I discovered more effective means against this original malady that caused so many complaints; against this malady which may be called by the general name of *Psora; i. e.*, against the internal itch disease with or without its attendant eruption on the skin. It then became manifest to me, through the aid afforded when using these medicines in similar chronic diseases, in which the patient was unable to show a like cause, that also these cases in which the patient remembered no infection of this kind were of necessity caused by a *Psora* with which he had been infected, perhaps, even in his cradle, or in some other way that had escaped his memory; and this often received corroboration on a more careful inquiry with the parents or aged relatives.

*So also, more lately, VON AUTENRIETH (in *Tübinger Blätter für Naturwissenschaft und Arzneikunde*, 2 vol., 2d part).

Most painstaking observations as to the aid afforded by the antipsoric remedies, which were added in the first of these eleven years, have taught me evermore how frequently not only the moderate, but also the more severe and the most severe, chronic diseases are of this origin. This observation taught me that not only most of the many cutaneous eruptions, which *Willan* distinguishes with such extreme care from one another, and which have received separate names, but also almost all adventitious formations, from the common wart on the finger up to the largest sarcomatous tumor, from the malformations of the finger-nails up to the swellings of the bones and the curvature of the spine, and many other softenings and deformities of the bones, both at an early and at a more advanced age, are caused by the *Psora*. So, also, frequent epistaxis, the accumulation of blood in the veins of the rectum and the anus, discharges of blood from the same (blind or flowing piles), hemoptysis, hematemesis, hematuria, and deficient as well as too frequent menstrual discharges, nightsweats of several years' duration, parchment-like dryness of the skin, diarrhœa of many years' standing, as well as permanent constipation and difficult evacuation of the bowels, long-continued erratic pains, convulsions occurring repeatedly for a number of years, chronic ulcers and inflammations, sarcomatous enlargements and tumors, emaciation, excessive sensitiveness as well as deficiencies in the senses of seeing, hearing, smelling, tasting and feeling; excessive as well as extinguished sexual desire, diseases of the mind and of the soul, from imbecility up to ecstacy, from melancholy up to raging insanity;

swoons and vertigo; the so-called diseases of the heart; abdominal complaints and all that is comprehended under hysteria and hypochondria—in short, thousands of tedious ailments of humaniiy called by pathology with various names, are, with few exceptions, true descendants of this many-formed *Psora* alone. I was thus instructed by my continued observations, comparisons and experiments in the last years that the ailments and infirmities of body and soul, which, in their manifest complaints, differ so radically, and which, with different patients, appear so very unlike (if they do not belong to the two venereal diseases, *syphilis* and *sycosis*) are but partial manifestations of the ancient miasma of leprosy and itch; *i. e.*, merely descendants of one and the same vast original malady, the almost innumerable symptoms of which form but one whole and are to be regarded and to be medicinally treated as the parts of one and the same disease in the same way as in a great epidemic of typhus fever. Thus, in the year 1813, one patient would be prostrated with only a few symptoms of this plague, a second patient showed only a few, but different ailments, while a third, fourth, etc., would complain of still other ailments belonging to this epidemic disease, while they were, nevertheless, all sick with one and the same pestilential fever, and the entire and complete image of the typhus fever reigning at the time could only be obtained by gathering together the symptoms of all, or at least of many of these patients. Then the one or two remedies* found to be homœopathic healed the

*In the typhus of 1813 *Bryonia* and *Rhus toxicodendron* were the specific remedies for all the patients.

whole epidemy, and therefore showed themselves specifically helpful with every patient, though the one might be suffering from symptoms differing from those of others, and almost all seemed to be suffering from different diseases.

Just so, only upon a *far larger* scale, it is with the *Psora*, this fundamental disease of so many chronic maladies, each of which seems to be essentially different from the others, but really is not, as may readily be seen from the agreement of several symptoms common to them which appear as the disease runs its course, and also from their being healed through the same remedy.

All chronic diseases of mankind, even those left to themselves, not aggravated by a perverted treatment, show, as said, such a constancy and perseverance, that as soon as they have developed and have not been thoroughly healed by the medical art, they evermore increase with the years, and during the whole of man's lifetime; and they cannot be diminished by the strength belonging even to the most robust constitution. Still less can they be overcome and extinguished Thus they never pass away of themselves, but increase and are aggravated even till death. They must therefore all have for their origin and foundation constant chronic miasms, whereby their parasitical existence in the human organism is enabled to continually rise and grow.

In Europe and also on other continents so far as is known, according to all investigations, only three chronic miasms are found, the diseases caused by which manifest themselves through local symptoms, and from which most, if not all, the chronic diseases originate; namely, first, SYPHILIS, which I have also called the *venereal chancre disease;* then SYCOSIS, or *the fig-wart disease*, and finally the chronic disease which lies at the foundation of the eruption of itch; *i. e.*, the PSORA; which I shall treat of first as the most important.

PSORA is that *most ancient*, *most universal*, *most destructive*, and yet *most misapprehended* chronic miasmatic disease which for many thousands of years has disfigured and tortured mankind, and which during the last centuries has become the mother of all the thousands of incredibly various (acute and) chronic (non-venereal) diseases, by which the whole civilized human race on the inhabited globe is being more and more afflicted.

PSORA is the *oldest* miasmatic chronic disease known to us. Just as tedious as syphilis and sycosis, and therefore not to be extinguished before the last breath of the longest human life, unless it is thoroughly cured, since not even the most robust constitution is able to destroy and extinguish it by its own proper strength, *Psora*, or the Itch disease, is beside this the *oldest* and *most hydra-headed* of all the chronic miasmatic diseases.

In the many thousands of years during which it may have afflicted mankind,—for the most ancient history of the most ancient people does not reach to its origin,—it has so much increased in the extent of its pathological manifestations—an extent which may to

---

† See Organon of the Healing Art, fifth edition, 1834, § 100 sqq.

some degree be explained by its increased development during such an inconceivable number of years in so many millions of organisms through which it has passed,—that its secondary symptoms are hardly to be numbered. And, if we except those diseases which have been created by a perverse medical practice or by deleterious labors in quicksilver, Lead, Arsenic, etc., which appear in the common pathology under a hundred proper names as supposedly separate and well-defined diseases (and also those springing from *syphilis* and the still rarer ones springing from *sycosis*), all the remaining natural chronic diseases, whether with names or without them, find in PSORA their real origin, their only source.

The oldest monuments of history which we possess show the *Psora* even then in great development. Moses* 3400 years ago pointed out several varieties. At that time and later on among the Israelites the dis-

---

*In Leviticus not only in the thirteenth chapter, but also (chap. 21, verse 20) where he speaks of the bodily defects which must not be found in a priest who is to offer sacrifice, malignant itch is designated by the word *garab*, which the Alexandrian translators (in the Septuagint) translated with *Psora agria*, but the Vulgate with *scabies jugis*. The talmudic interpreter, Jonathan, explained it as *dry itch spread over the body;* while the expression, *yalephed*, is used by Moses for *lichen*, *tetter*, *herpes* (see M. Rosenmueller, *Scholia in Levit.*, p. II., *edit. sec.*, p. 124) The commentators in the so-called English Bible-work also agree with this definition, Calmet, among others, saying: "Leprosy is similar to an inveterate itch with violent itching." The ancients also mention the peculiar, characteristic *voluptuous* itching which attended itch then as now, while after the scratching a painful burning follows; among others Plato, who calls itch *glykypikron*, while Cicero marks the *dulcedo* of *scabies*.

ease seems to have mostly kept the external parts of the body for its chief seat. This was also true of the malady as it prevailed in uncultivated Greece, later in Arabia and, lastly in Europe, during the Middle Ages. The different names which were given by different nations to the more or less malignant varieties of leprosy (the external symptom of *Psora*), which in many ways deformed the external parts of the body, do not concern us and do not affect the matter, since the nature of this miasmatic itching eruption always remained essentially the same.

The occidental *Psora*, which, during the Middle Ages, had raged in Europe for several centuries under the form of malignant erysipelas (called *St. Anthony's Fire*), reassumed the form of leprosy through the leprosy which was brought back by the returning crusaders in the thirteenth century. And though it thus spread in Europe even more than before (for in the year 1226 there were in France alone 2,000 houses for the reception of lepers), this Psora, which now raged as a dreadful eruption, found at least an external alleviation in the means conducive to cleanliness, which also were brought by the crusaders from the Orient, namely, the (cotton? linen?) shirts before unknown in Europe, and the more frequent use of warm baths. Through both of those means, as well as through the more exquisite diet and refinement in the mode of living introduced by increased cultivation, the external horrors of the Psora within the space of several centuries were at last so far moderated that, at the end of the fifteenth century, it appeared only in the form of the common eruption of itch, just at the time when the other miasmatic chronic disease, *syphilis*, began (in 1493) to raise its dreadful head.

Thus this eruption, externally reduced in cultivated countries to a common itch, could be much more easily removed from the skin through various means, so that with the medicinal external treatmènt since introduced, especially in the middle and higher classes, through baths, washes and ointments of sulphur and lead, and by preparations of copper, zinc and mercury, the external manifestations of *Psosa* on the skin were often so quickly suppressed, and are so now, that in most cases, either of children or of grown persons, the history of itch infection may remain undiscovered.

But the state of mankind was not improved thereby; in many respects it grew far worse. For, although in ancient times the eruption of Psora appearing as leprosy was very troublesume to those suffering from it, owing to the lancinating pains in and the violent itching all around the tumors and scabs, the rest of the body enjoyed a fair share of general health. This was owing to the obstinately persistent eruption on the skin, which served as a substitute for the internal Psora. And what is of more importance, the horrible and disgusting appearance of the lepers made such a terrible impression on healthy people that they dreaded even their approach, so that the seclusion of most of these patients, and their separation in leper hospitals, kept them apart from other human society and infection from them was thus limited and comparatively rare.

In consequence of the very much milder form of the *Psora* during the fourteenth and fifteenth centuries, when it appeared as itch, the few pustules appearing after infection made but little show and could easily be concealed. Nevertheless they were scratched continually because of their unbearable itching, and thus the fluid was diffused around, and the psoric miasma was communicated more certainly and more easily to many other persons the more it was concealed; for the things rendered unclean by the psoric fluid infected the persons who unwittingly touched them, and thus contaminated far more persons than the lepers, who, on account of their horrible appearance, were carefully avoided.

PSORA has thus become the *most infectious* and ***most general*** of all the chronic miasmas. For the miasm has usually been communicated to others before the one from whom it emanates has asked for or received any external repressive remedy against his itching eruption (lead-water, ointment of the white precipitate of mercury), and without confessing that he had an eruption of itch, often even without knowing it himself; yea, without even the physician's or surgeon's knowing the exact nature of the eruption, which has been repressed by the lotion of lead, etc.

It may well be conceived that the poorer and lower classes, who allow the itch to spread on their skin for a long time, until they become an abomination to all around them, and are compelled to use something to remove it, must have in the meanwhile infected many.

Mankind, therefore, is worse off from the change in the external form of the *Psora*,—from leprosy down to the eruption of itch—not only because this is less visible and more secret and therefore more frequently infectious, but also especially because the *Psora*, now mitigated externally into a mere itch and on that account more generally spread, nevertheless still retains unchanged its original dreadful nature. Now, after being more easily repressed, the disease grows all the more unperceived within, and so, in the last three centuries, after the destruction* of its chief symptom (the

*The external eruption of itch may not only be driven away by the faulty practices of physicians and quacks, but unfortunately it not unfrequently of its own accord withdraws from the skin (see below, *e. g.*, in the observation of the older physicians, Nos. 9, 17, 26, 36, 50, 58, 61, 64, 65). *Syphilis* and *sycosis* both have an advantage over the itch disease in this, that the chancre (or bubo) in the one and the fig-wart in the other never leave the external parts until they have been either mischievously destroyed through external repressive remedies or have been in a rational manner removed through the simultaneous internal cure of the whole disease. The venereal disease cannot, therefore, break out so long as the chancre is not artificially destroyed by external applications, nor can the secondary ailments of sycosis break out so long as the fig-wart has not been destroyed by faulty practice; for these local symptoms, which act as substitutes for the internal disease, remain standing even until the end of man's life, and prevent the breaking out of the internal disease. It is, therefore, just as easy to heal them then, even in their whole extent, *i. e.*, thoroughly, through their specific internal medicines, which need only to be continued until these local symptoms (chancre and fig-wart), which are in their nature *unchangeable* except through artificial external application, are thoroughly healed. Then we may be quite certain that we have thoroughly cured the internal disease, *i. e.*, *syphilis* and *sycosis*.

This good feature *Psora* has lost in the present more and more mitigated nature of its chief symptom, which has changed from leprosy to itch in the last three centuries. The eruption of itch by no means remains as persistently in its place on the skin as the chancre and fig-wart. Even if the eruption of itch has not (as is

external skin eruption) it plays the sad rôle of causing innumerable secondary symptoms, *i. e.*, it originates a legion of chronic diseases, the source of which physicians neither surmise nor unravel, and which, therefore, they can no more cure than they could cure the original disease when accompanied by its cutaneous eruption; but these chronic diseases, as daily experience shows, were necessarily aggravated by the multitude of their faulty remedies.

---

nearly always the case) been driven away from the skin through the faulty practices of physicians and quacks by means of desiccating washes, sulphur ointments, drastic purgatives or cupping, it frequently disappears, as we say, *of itself*, *i. e.*, through causes which are not noticed. It often disappears through some unlucky physical or psychical occurrence, through a violent fright, through continual vexations, deeply-affecting grief, through catching a severe cold, or through a cold temperature (see below, observation 67); through cold, lukewarm and warm river baths or mineral baths, by a fever arising from any cause, or through a different acute disease (*e. g.*, smallpox; see below, observation 39); through persistent diarrhœa, sometimes also perhaps through a peculiar want of activity in the skin, and the results in such a case are just as mischievous as if the eruption had been driven away externally by the irrational practice of a physician. The secondary ailments of the internal *Psora* and any one of the innumerable chronic diseases flowing from this origin will then break out sooner or later.

But let no one think that the *Psora*, which has been thus mitigated in its local symptom, its cutaneous eruption, differs materially from ancient leprosy. Even leprosy, when not inveterate, could in ancient times not seldom be driven from the skin by cold baths or by repeated dipping in a river and through warm mineral baths (see below, No. 35); but also then the evil effects resulting were as little regarded as the more modern physicians regard the acute diseases and the insidious maladies which do not fail to develop sooner or later from the indwelling *Psora* when an eruption of the present itch disease has disappeared of itself or has been violently driven away.

So great a flood of numberless nervous troubles, painful ailments, spasms, ulcers (cancers), adventitious formations, dyscrasias, paralyses, consumptions and cripplings of soul, mind and body were never seen in ancient times when the *Psora* mostly confined itself to its dreadful cutaneous symptom, leprosy. Only during the last few centuries has mankind been flooded with these infirmities, owing to the causes just mentioned.*

It was thus that PSORA became the *most universal* mother of chronic diseases.

The *Psora*, which is now so easily and so rashly robbed of its ameliorating cutaneous symptom, the eruption of itch, which acts vicariously for the internal disease, has been producing within the last three hundred years more and more secondary symptoms, and, indeed, so many that at least *seven-eighths* of all the chronic maladies spring from it as their only source,

*That the drinking of warm coffee and Chinese tea, which has spread so generally in the last two centuries, and which has so largely increased the irritability of the muscular fibre as well as the excessive excitability of the nerves, has further augmented the tendency of this period to a multitude of chronic diseases, and has thus aided the *Psora*, I least of all *can doubt*, as I have made prominent, perhaps too prominent, the part which coffee takes with respect to the bodily and mental sufferings of humanity in my little work on "The Effects of Coffee" (*Die Wirkungen des Kaffee's*, Leipzig, 1803). This, perhaps undue, prominence given was owing to the fact that I had not then as yet discovered the chief source of chronic diseases in the *Psora*. Only in connection with the excessive use of coffee and tea, which both offer palliatives for several symptoms of *Psora*, could *Psora* spread such innumerable, such obstinate chronic sufferings among mankind; for Psora alone could not have produced this effect.

while the *remaining eighth* springs from *syphilis* and *sycosis*, or from a complication of two of these three miasmatic chronic diseases, or (which is rare) from a complication of all three of them. Even *syphilis*, which on account of its easy curability yields to the smallest dose of the best preparation of Mercury, and *sycosis*, which on account of the slight difficulty in its cure through a few doses of Thuja and Nitric acid in alternation, only pass into a tedious malady difficult to cure when they are complicated with Psora. Thus PSORA *is among all diseases the one which is most misapprehended, and, therefore, has been medically treated in the worst and most injurious manner.*

It is incredible to what an extent modern physicians of the common school have sinned against the welfare of humanity, since, with scarcely an exception, teachers of medicine and the more prominent modern physicians and medical writers have laid down the rule and taught it as an infallible theorem that: "Every eruption of itch is merely a local ailment of the skin, in which ailment the remaining organism takes no part at all, so that it may and must be driven away from the skin at any time and without any scruple, through local applications of sulphur ointment or of the yet more active ointment of Jasser, through sulphur fumigations, by solutions of lead and zinc, but most quickly by the precipitates of mercury. If the eruption is once removed from the skin everything is well and the person is restored and the whole disease removed. Of course, if the eruption is neglected and allowed to spread upon the skin, then it may eventually turn out that the malignant matter may find opportunity to insinuate itself through the absorbent vessels into the mass of humors and thus to corrupt the blood, the humors and the health. Then, indeed, man may finally be afflicted with ailments from these malignant humors, though these might soon again be removed from the body by purgatives and abluents; but through prompt removal of the eruption from the skin all sequelæ are prevented and the internal body remains entirely healthy."

These horrible untruths have not only been, and are still being taught, but they are also being carried out in practice. The consequence is that at the present day the patients in all the most celebrated hospitals, even in those countries and cities that seem most enlightened, as well as the pr vate itch-patients of the lower and higher classes, the patients in all the penitentiaries and orphan asylums, in other civil and military hospitals, wherever such eruptions are found—in short, the innumerable multitude of patients, without exception, are treated, not only by physicians unknown to fame but by all, even those *most celebrated*, with the above mentioned external remedies,* using

---

* Then, as these gentlemen dream in their perverted minds, in which they have disposed of the nature of this most important disease in their arbitrary way and without consulting nature, then these frivolous gentlemen assure us, the matter of the itch has not yet had time to penetrate inwardly and to be received by the absorbent vessels to the detriment of the whole mass of humors. But how then, Oh conscientious men! if even the first little pustule of itch with its unbearable voluptuous itching, forcing a man irresistibly to scratch, and with the following burning pain, is *in every case and every time* the proof of a universal itch-disease which has been previously developed in the interior of the whole organism, as we shall see below? How then, if in accordance with this fact

perhaps at the same time large doses of flowers of sulphur, and strong purgatives (to cleanse the body, as they say). These physicians think that the more quickly these eruptions are driven from the skin the better. Then they dismiss the patients from their treatment as cured, with brazen assurance and the delaration that everything is now all right,* without regarding or being willing to notice the ailments which sooner or later are sure to follow; *i. e.*, the *Psora* which shows itself from within in a thousand different diseases.† If the deceived wretches then soonor or later return with the malady following *unavoidably* on

---

any external repression of the itch-eruption can not only do nothing toward alleviating the internal general disease, but rather as thousands of facts go to prove, compel it to develop and break forth quickly into innumerable, different, acute sufferings, or gradully into chronic sufferings, which make mankind so help less and miserable? Can you then heal these? Experience says no; you cannot do it.

*In some vigorous itch patients the vital force, following the law of nature on which its rests (her instinct showing more wisdom than the intelligence of her destroyers), after some weeks, drives back to the skin the eruption seemingly destroyed by itch ointments and purgatives; the patient returns to the hospital and the mischievous destruction of the eruption, by means of ointments and lotions of solutions of Lead and Zinc, is renewed. I have seen in military hospitals this eruption thus destroyed in an irrational and cruel manner three times in succession within a few months, while the quack who applied the ointment pretended that the patient must have been infected anew with itch three times in this short period, which was really impossible.

† I wrote this six years ago, but even at this day the physicians of the old school continue to act and teach with the same criminal negligence. In this most important medical affair they have up to this day not become the least bit wiser or more humane.

such a treatment; *e. g.*, with swellings, obstinate pains in one part or another, with hypochondriac or hysterical troubles, gout, consumption, tubercular phthisis, continual or spasmodic asthma, blindness, deafness, paralysis, caries of the bones, ulcers (cancer), spasms, hemorrhages, diseases of the mind and soul, etc., the physicians smagine that they have before them something entirely new and treat it again and again according to the old routine of their therapeutics in a useless and hurtful manner, directing their medicines against phantom diseases; *i. e.*, against causes invented by them for the ailments as they appear, until the patient, after many years' suffering continually aggravated, is at last freed from their hands by death, the end of all earthly maladies.*

The older physicians were more conscientious in this matter and observed with less prejudice. They saw clearly and became convinced that innumerable ailments and the most severe chronic diseases follow the destruction of the itch-eruption from the skin. And since this experience compelled them to assume the existence of an internal disease, in every case of itch

* By accident (for they cannot give any but a feigned reason for their action) they found out a refuge which temporarily often alleviates the sufferings of their patients when they cannot do anything at home with their prescriptions against the unknown disease; that is, they send him to some sulphur bath or other where the patients often get rid of a small part of their *Psora*, and thus are also at the first use of the baths for a time relieved of their chronic disease; but afterwards they fall back into the same or a kindred ailment, and the repetition of the bath then avails little or nothing, because the cure of a developed *Psora* requires a far more adequate treatment than the impetuous use of such baths.

they endeavor to extirpate this internal malady by means of a multitude of internal remedies, as good as their therapeutics afforded. It was, indeed, but a useless endeavor, because the true method of healing, which it could only be the prerogative of Homœopathy to discover, was unknown to them. Nevertheless this sincere endeavor was praiseworthy, since it was founded on an appreciation of the great internal disease present, together with the eruption of itch, which internal disease it was necessary to remove. This prevented their reliance on the mere local destruction of the itch from the skin, as practiced by modern physicians, who think that they cannot quickly enough drive it away—as if it were a mere external disease of the skin—without regarding the great injuries attending such a course. The older physicians, on the other hand, have warningly laid these injuries before our eyes in their writings, giving thousands of examples.

The observations of those honest men are too startling to be rejected contemptuously, or ignored by conscientious men.

I shall here adduce some of these numerous observations handed down to us, which I might increase by an equal number of my own if the former were not already abundantly sufficient to show with what fury the internal *Psora* manifests itself when the external local symptom which serves to assuage the internal malady is hastily removed. They also show that it must be a matter of conscience for the physician who loves his fellow-man to direct all his endeavors to cure, first of all, the internal malady, whereby the cutaneous eruption will at the same time be removed and destroyed and all the subsequent innumerable life-long chronic sufferings springing from the *Psora* be prevented or, if they are already embittering the life of the patient, be cured.

The diseases, partly acute but chiefly chronic, springing from such a one-sided destruction of the chief skin-symptom (eruption and itching) which acts vicariously and assuages the internal *Psora* (which destruction is erroneously called "*Driving the itch into the body*") are innumerable; as manifold as the peculiarities of bodily constitutions and of the outer world which modifies them.

A brief survey of the manifold misfortunes resulting thence is given by the experienced and honest LUDWIG CHRISTIAN JUNCKER in his *Dissertatio de Damno ex Scabie Repulsa*, *Halle*, 1750, p. 15–18. He observed that with young people of a sanguine temperament the suppression of itch is followed by phthisis, and with persons in general who are of a sanguine temperament it is followed by piles, hemorrhoidal colic and renal gravel; with persons of sanguino-choleric temperament by swellings of the inguinal glands, stiffening of the joints and malignant ulcers (called in German *Todenbrüche*); with fat persons by a suffocating catarrh and mucous consumption; also by inflammatory fever, acute pleurisy and inflammation of the lungs. He further states that in autopsies the lungs have been found indurated and full of cysts containing pus; also other indurations, swellings of the bones and ulcers have been seen to follow the suppression of an eruption. Phlegmatic persons in consequence of such suppressions suffered chiefly from dropsy; the menses were delayed, and when the itch was driven away during their flow, they were changed into a monthly hemoptysis. Persons inclined to melancholy were sometimes made insane by such repression; if they were pregnant the fœtus was usually killed. Sometimes the suppression of the itch causes sterility,* in nursing women the milk is generally lacking, the menses disappear prematurely; in older women the uterus becomes ulcerated, attended with deep, burning pains, with wasting away (cancer of the womb).

His experiences were frequently confirmed by the observations† of others, as *e. g.* with reference to:

---

*A pregnant Jewess had the itch on her hands and drove it away in the eighth month of her pregnancy so that it might not be seen during the period of her delivery. Three days afterwards she was delivered and the lochial discharge did not appear and she was seized with a high fever; since that time for seven years she had been sterile and had suffered from leucorrhœa Then she became poor and had to walk a great distance barefooted; hereupon the itch again appeared and she thus lost her leucorrhœa and her other hysteric affections; she became again pregnant and was safely delivered (*Juncker*, ibid.)

† When writing the first edition of the Chronic Diseases, I was not as yet acquainted with **Autenrieth's** *Versuche fuer die prakt. Heilkunde aus den Klinishen Anstalten von Tubingen*, 1808. But I saw on examining the work, that what he says about diseases following the driving away of itch through local applications is only a confirmation of what I had already found with the other hundred writers. He also had observed that the external driving away of itch was followed by ulcers on the feet, pulmonary consumption, hysterical chlorosis, with various menstrual irregularities; white swelling of the knee, dropsy of the joints, epilepsy, amaurosis, with obscured cornea; glaucoma with complete amaurosis; mental derangement, paralysis, apoplexy and curvature of the neck; these he erroneously attributed to the

Asthma, Lentilius *Miscell. med. pract.* Tom. I., p. 176. **Fr. Hoffmann** *Abhandlung v. d. Kinderkrankheiten*, Frft., 1741, p. 104. **Detharding** in *Append. ad Ephem. Nat. Cur. Dec.* III., *ann 5 et, 6 et in obs. parallel. ad obs. 58.* **Binninger,** *Obs. Cent.* V., *obs. 88.* **Morgagni,** *de sedibus et caus. morb. Epist.*, XIV. 35. *Acta Nat. Cur. Tom.* V. *obs.* 47. **J. Juncker,** *Consp. ther. spec. tab.* 31. **F. H. L. Muzell,** *Wahrnehm. Samml.* II. *Cas. 8.*[1] **J. Fr. Gmelin** in **Gesner's** *Samml. v. Beob. V.* S. 21.[2] **Hundertmark-Zieger** *Dissert. de scabie artificiale, Lips.*

---

ointments alone. But his own slow local driving away of the eruption by means of sulphuret of potash and soft soap, which he in vain calls *healing* it, is in no way better. Just as if his treatment were anything else than a local driving away of the eruption from the skin! Of any true cure he knows just as little as the other Allopaths, for he writes: "It is, of course, absurd to endeavor to cure itch (scab) by internal remedies." No! it is not only absurd, but even wretched to undertake to cure an internal itch-disease which cannot be cured by any *local* application, through any but *internal* means, which alone can cure the disease *thoroughly and with certainty*.

[1] A man 30 to 40 years of age had been affiicted with the itch a long time before, and it had been driven away by ointments; from which time he had become more and more asthmatic. His respiration became at last, even when not in motion, very short and extremely labored, emitting at the same time a continuous hissing sound, but attended with only little coughing. He was ordered an injection of one drachm of squills, and to take internally 3 grains of squills. But by mistake he took the drachm of squills internally. He was near losing his life with an indescribable nausea and retching. Soon after this the itch appeared again on his hands, his feet and his whole body in great abundance, and by this means the asthma was at once removed.

[2] The violent asthma was combined with general swelling and fever.

1758, p. 32.[3] **Beireis—Stammen.** *Diss. de causis cur imprimis plebs scabie laboret.* Helmst., 1792, p. 26.[4] **Pelargus** (*Storch*) *Obs. clin. Jahrg.*, 1722, p. 435 *n* 438.[5] *Breslauer Sammlung v. Jahre*, 1727, p. 293.[6] **Riedlin,** the father, *Obs. Cent.* II., *obs.* 90. Augsburg, 1691.[7]

Suffocating Catarrh, Ehrenfr. Hagendorn, *hist. med. phys.*

---

[3] A man of 32 years had the itch driven away by sulphur ointment, and he suffered for eleven months from the most violent asthma until by drinking birch-juice the eruption was brought back on the twenty-third day.

[4] A student was seized with the itch just as he was going to dance, on which account he had it driven out by a practitioner with sulphur ointment. But soon after, he was attacked by such a severe asthma that he could only draw breath by throwing his head back, and was almost suffocated during the attacks. After thus wrestling with death for an hour, he would cough up little cartilaginous pieces which would ease him for a very short time. Having returned home to Osterode he suffered continually for two years of this disease, being attacked about ten times a day, which could not even be mitigated through the help of his physician, **Beireis.**

[5] A boy of 13 years having suffered from his childhood with *tinea capitis* had his mother remove it for him, but he became very sick within eight or ten days, suffering with asthma, violent pains in the limbs, back and knee, which were not relieved until an eruption of itch broke out over his whole body a month later.

[6] *Tinea capitis* in a little girl was driven away by purgatives and other medicines, but the child was attacked with oppression of the chest, cough and great lassitude. It was not until she stopped taking the medicines, and the *tinea* broke out again, that she recovered her cheerfulness and this, indeed, quickly.

[7] A boy of 5 years suffered for a long time from itch, and when this was driven away by a salve it left behind a severe melancholy with a cough.

Cent. I., *hist* 8, 9.[8] **Pelargus,** *Obs. clin. Jahrg.*, 1723 p. 15.[9]

Suffocations from Asthma, Joh. Phil. Brendel, *Consilia med.*, *Frft.*, 1615, *Cons.* 73. *Ephem. Nat. Cur.*, Ann. II., obs. 313. **Wilh. Fabr. V. Hilden,** *Obs. Cent.* III., *Obs.* 39.[10] **Ph. R. Vicat,** *Obs. Pract.*, *obs.* 35, *Vitoduri*, 1780.[11] **J. J. Waldschmid,** *Opera*, p. 244.[12]

---

[8] Owing to *tinea capitis*, which had been driven off by rubbing with almond oil, there arose an excessive lassitude of all the limbs, headache on one side, loss of appetite, asthma, waking up at night with suffocating catarrh, with severe rattling and whistling on the chest and convulsive twisting of the limbs, as if about to die, and hematuria. When the tinea broke out again, he recovered from all these ailments.

A 3-year-old girl had the itch, for several weeks; when this was driven out by an ointment she was seized the next day by a suffocating catarrh with snoring, and with numbness and coldness of the whole body, from which she did not recover until the itch reappeared.

[9] A girl of twelve years had the itch with which she had frequently suffered, driven away from the skin by an ointment, when she was seized with an acute fever with suffocative catarrh, asthma and swelling, and afterward with pleurisy. Six days afterward, having taken an internal medicine containing sulphur, the itch again appeared and all the ailments, excepting the swelling, disappeared; but after twenty-four days the itch again dried up, which was followed by a new inflammation in the chest with pleurisy and vomiting.

[10] The dyspnœa of a youth, 20 years, caused by the driving away of itch was so great that he could not get any breath, and his pulse was hardly perceptible, in consequence of which he suffocated.

[11] A moist herpes on the left upper arm of a youth of 19 years was finally locally removed by many external applications. But soon after, there ensued a periodical asthma which was suddenly increased by a lengthy foot-tour in the heat of summer, even to suffocation, with a puffed up bluish-red face and quick, weak, uneven pulse.

[12] The dyspnœa from the driven out itch came on very suddenly, and the patient was suffocated.

Asthma with General Swelling. Waldschmid, ibid. **Hoechstetter,** *Obs. Dec.* III., *obs.* 7 Frft. et Lips, 1674, p. 248. **Pelargus,** *Obs. Clin. Jahrg.*, 1723, p. 504.[13] **Riedlin,** the father, *Obs. Cent.* II., *obs.* 91.[14]

Asthma with Dropsy of the Chest. Storch *in Act. Nat. Cur. Tom.* V., *obs.* 147. **Morgagni,** *de sed. et causis morb.* XVI., Art. 34.[15] **Richard,** *Recueil d' observ. de Med. Tom.* III., p. 308, à Paris, 1772. **Hagendorn,** as above, Cent. II., hist. 15.[16]

Pleurisy and Inflammation in the Chest, Pelargus, as above, p. 10.[17] **Hagendorn,** as above, *Cent.* III., *hist.* 58. **Giseke,**

---

[13] A 5-year-old girl had had for some time large itch vesicles on the hands, which dried up of themselves. Shortly after, she became sleepy and tired and was seized with dyspnœa. The following day the asthma continued and her abdomen became distended.

[14] A 50-year-old farmer, who had been long tortured with the itch, while he was driving it out by external applications, was seized with a dyspnœa, a loss of appetite and a swelling of the whole body.

[15] A girl in Bologna drove away the itch with an ointment and was seized with the most severe asthma without fever. After two blood-lettings her strength decreased so much and the asthma was so much augmented that she died on the following day. The whole chest was filled with bluish water, also the pericardium.

[16] A girl of 9 years with the *tinea capitis* had it driven away, when she was seized with a lingering fever, a general swelling and dyspnœa; when the *tinea* broke out again she recovered.

[17] A man of 46 drove out his itch with a sulphur ointment. Thereupon he was seized with inflammation in the chest, with bloody expectoration, dyspnœa and great anguish. The following day the heat and the anguish became almost unbearable and the pains in the chest increased on the third day. Then sweat broke out. After fourteen days the itch broke out again and he felt better. But he had a relapse, the itch dried up again, and he died on the thirteenth day after the relapse.

Hamb. Abhandl., p. 310. **Richard,** as above. **Pelargus,** as above. *Jahrg.*, 1721, p. 23 and 114,[18] and *Jahrg.*, 1723, p. 29,[19] also in *Jahrg.*, 1722, p. 459.[20] **Sennert,** *praxis med. lib.* II., *P.* III., *Cap.* 6, p. 380. **Jerzembsky,** *Diss. Scabies salubris in hydrope*, Halae, 1777.[21] **Karl Wenzel,** *Die Nachkrankheiten von zurückgetretener Krätze*, Bamb., 1826, p. 49.[22]

Pleurisy and Cough, Pelargus, as above, Jahrg., 1722, p. 79.[23]

Severe Cough, Richard, as above. **Juncker,** *Conspect. med. theor. et pract. tab.*, 76. **Hundertmark,** as above, p. 23.[23*]

Hemoptysis, Phil. Georg. Schroeder, *Opusc.* II., p. 322. **Richard,** as above. **Binninger,** Obs. Cent. V., obs. 88.

Hemoptysis and Consumption. Chn. Max. Spener, *Diss. de egro febri maligni phthisi complicata laborante*, Giess,

---

[18] A thin man died of inflammation in the chest and other ailments twenty days after driving out the itch.

[19] A boy of 7 years whose *tinea capitis* and itch dried up, died after four days from an acute fever and asthma accompanied by expectoration.

[20] A youth who removed his itch with a lead ointment, died four days afterward of a disease of the chest.

[21] A general dropsy was quickly cured by a return of the itch, but when this was suppressed by a severe cold, pleurisy supervened and death ensued in three days.

[22] A young peasant was attacked with acute fever, with pleurisy and dyspnœa, six days after driving out an eruption of itch with sulphur ointment.

[23] A school boy of 13 years was seized with cough and stitches in the chest when his itch dried up. These ailments disappeared when the itch broke out again.

[23*] A man of 36 years had the itch removed sixteen months ago by an ointment of lead and mercury; he suffered since from a whooping cough accompanied by great anguish.

1699.[24] **Baglio,** *Opera*, p. 215. **Sicelius,** *Praxis casual. Exerc.* III., *Cas.* I., Frft. et Lips, 1743.[25] **Morgagni,** as above, XXI., *Art.* 32.[26] **Unzers,** *Arzt* C C C., p. 508.[27] **Karl Wenzel,** as above, p. 32.

Collection of Pus in the Chest. **F. A. Waitz,** *Medic. Chirurg. Aufsätz Th.* I., p. 114, 115.[28] **Preval,** in the *Journal de Médec.*, LXI., p. 491.

Cysts of Pus in the Intestines, Krause. **Schubert,** *Diss. de scabie humana.* Lips. 1779, p. 23.[29]

Great Degeneration of a Great Part of the Intestines. **J. H. Schulze,** in *Act. Nat. Cur. Tom.*, 1 *obs.*, 231.[30]

---

[24] A youth of 18 years had the itch, which he finally drove away with a black-looking lotion. A few days after he was seized with chills and heat, lassitude, oppression of the heart, headache, nausea, violent thirst, cough and difficulty in breathing; he expectorated blood, commenced to speak deliriously, his face was deadly pale and sunken, the urine was deep red without sediment.

[25] An eruption of itch in a youth of 18 years driven out by a mercurial plaster.

[26] Itch which disappeared from the skin of itself was followed by a lingering fever and fatal expectoration of pus; at the autopsy the left lung was found full of pus.

[27] A robust looking candidate for the ministry who was about to preach in a few days and therefore wished to free himself from his old itch, rubbed himself one day with itch ointment and in a few hours, soon after noon, he passed away with anxiety, dyspnœa and tenesmus; the autopsy showed that the whole of the lungs was filled with liquid pus.

[28] Empyema followed the driving away, through external means, of an eruption of itch which had come out a few years before, and appeared especially in March and April.

[29] A young man who had been warned by (the good physician and) Prof. Krause against the use of sulphur ointment for the reappearing itch, did not follow his advice, but rubbed himself with it, when he died of constipation. In his body, at the autopsy, were found sacs of pus in his abdominal viscera.

[30] Also the diaphragm and the liver were diseased.

Degeneration of the Brain. Dimenbrock, *Obs. et Curat. med., obs.* 60. **Bonet,** *Sepulchretum anat., Sect.* IV., *obs.* 1, § 1[31] and § 2.[32] **J. H. Schulze,** as above.

Hydrocephalus, *Acta helvet.*, V., p. 190.

Ulcers in the Stomach. L. Chn. Juncker, *Diss. de scabie repulsa*, Halle, 1750, p. 16.[33]

Sphacelus of the Stomach and Duodenum. Hundertmark, as above, p. 29.[34]

General Dropsical Swelling.[35]

Dropsy of the Chest. Hessler in **Karl Wenzel,** as above, p. 100 and 102.

---

[31] A little prince of two years had his *tinea capitis* driven away; in consequence, after his death, much bloody water was found under his skull.

[32] In a woman who had driven out the *tinea* by a lotion, one-half of the brain was found putrefied and filled with yellow humor.

[33] A man of rank, of a cholerico-sanguine temperament, was afflicted with gouty pains of the abdomen and pains as from gravel. After the removal of the gout through various remedies the itch broke out, which he drove out through a desiccating bath of tan-bark; an ulcer formed on his stomach, which, as the autopsy showed, hastened his death.

[34] A boy of 7 weeks and a youth of 18 years died very suddenly from an itch driven out through a sulphur ointment. At the autopsy, in the case of the infant, the upper part of the stomach immediately below the orifice was found destroyed by gangrene, and in the second case that part of the duodenum into which the biliary duct and the pancreatic duct empty was found similarly diseased. A similar fatal inflammation of the stomach from driven-out itch, in *Morgagni*, as above, LV., art. 11.

[35] Of this, innumerable cases are found in a number of writers, of which I only desire to mention the one reported in **J. D. Fick,** *Exercitatio med. de scabie retropulsa*, Halle, 1710, § 6, where an eruption of itch, driven out by application of mercury, left behind it general dropsy, which was only mitigated by the re-appearance of the eruption.

The author of the book *Epidemion lib.* 5, No. 4, who gives his

Dropsy of the Abdomen, Richard, as above, and with several other observers.

Swelling of the Scrotum (in boys). **Fr. Hoffman,** *Med. rat. syst.*, III., p. 175.

Red Swelling of the Whole Body. Lentilius, *Misc. med. pract.*, Part I., p. 176.

Jaundice. Baldinger, *Krankheiten ein. Armee*, p. 226. **Joh. Rud. Camerarius,** *Memorab. Cent.*, X., § 65.

Swelling of the Parotid Glands. Barette, in the *Journal de Méd.*, XVIII., p. 169.

Swelling of the Cervical Glands, Pelargus, as above, **Jahrg.,** 1723, p. 593.[36] **Unzer,** *Arzt.*, Part VI., *St.*, 301.[37]

Obscuration of the Eyes and Presbyopia, Fr. Hoffman, *Consult. med.*, 1 Cas. 50.[38]

---

name as **Hippocrates,** first mentions the sad result of such a case, where an Athenian was seized by a violently itching eruption, spread over the whole body and especially over the genital organs; he expelled it by the use of the warm baths on the island of Melos, but died of the resulting dropsy.

[36]A boy of 8 or 9 years, who had been shortly before healed of *tinea*, showed many swellings of the glands of the neck, by which his neck was drawn crooked and stiff.

[37]A youth of 14 years had the itch in June, 1761. He rubbed with a gray ointment and the itch passed away. Upon this the glands behind both of his ears swelled up; the swelling on the left ear passed away of itself, but the right one in five months became monstrously enlarged and about August began to pain him. All the glands of the neck were swollen. On the outside the large gland was full of hard knots and without sensitiveness, but internally there was an obtuse pain, especially at night; at the same time he suffered from dyspnœa and obstructed deglutition. All means used to produce suppuration were in vain; it became so large that the patient was suffocated in the year 1762.

[38]A girl of 13 years was seized with the itch, especially on the limbs, in the face and on the pudenda; this was finally driven away

Inflammation of the Eyes, G. W. Wedel. Snetter, *Diss.* **de Ophthalmia,** Jen., 1710. **Hallmann,** in *Kœnigl. Vetenskaps Handl.* f. A. X., p. 210.[39] **G. Chph. Schiller,** *de scabie humida*, p. 42, Erford., 1747.

Cataract, Chn. Gottlieb Ludwig, *Advers. med.* II., p. 157.[40]

Amaurosis, Northof, *Diss. de scabie*, Gotting., 1792, p. 10.[41] **Chn. G. Ludwig,** as above.[42] **Sennert,** *prax. lib.* III., *Sect.* 2, *Cap* 44. **Trecourt,** *chirurg. Wahrnehmungen*, p. 173., Leipz., 1777. **Fabricius ab Hilden,** *Cent.* II., *obs.* 39.[43]

---

by ointments of zinc and sulphur, whereupon she gradually became weak of sight. Little dark bodies floated before her eyes, and these could also be seen from without floating in the aqueous humor of the anterior chamber of the eye. At the same time she could not recognize small bodies except with spectacles. The pupils were dilated.

[39]A girl had a violent eruption of itch on the legs, with large ulcers in the bend of the knee. Being attacked with smallpox the itch was suppressed. This induced a humid inflammation of the white of the eye and of the eyelids, with itching and suppuration of the same, and the vision of dark bodies floating before her eyes; this lasted for two years. Then for three days she put on the stockings of a child afflicted with the itch. On the last day a fever broke out, with dry cough, tension in the chest, with inclination to vomit. On the following day the fever and the tension of the chest diminished and a sweat broke out, which increased until erysipelas broke out on both legs, and on the following day these passed over into the real itch. The eyes then improved.

[40]A man whose itch had been driven off, but who was of robust constitution, was seized with cataract.

[41]From itch expelled by external application there arose amaurosis, which passed away when the eruption re-appeared on the skin.

[42]A vigorous man, when the itch had been expelled from the skin, was seized with amaurosis and remained blind to an advanced age.

[43]Amaurosis from the same cause, with terrible headache.

Deafness. Thore in *Capelle, Journal de Santé*, Tom. I. **Daniel,** *Syst. aegritud.* II., p. 228. **Ludwig,** as above.

Inflammation of the Bowels, Hundertmark. *Diss. de scabie artificiali, Lips.* 1758, p. 29.

Pile's, Hemorrhoids, *Acta helvet.* V., p. 192.[44] **Daniel,** *Syst. aegritud.* II., p. 245.[45]

Abdominal Complaints, Fr. Hoffmann, *Med. rat. syst.* III., p. 177.[46]

Diabetes (Mellitaria), *Comment. Lips.* XIV., p. 365. *Eph. Nat. Cur. Dec.* II., *ann.* 10, p. 162. **C. Weber,** *Obs.* f. I., p. 26.

Suppression of Urine, Sennert, Prax. lib. 3, p. 8. **Morgagni,** as above, XLI., *art.* 2.[47]

Erysipelas, Unzer *Artz Th.* V., St. 301.[48]

Discharges of acrid humors. Fr. Hoffman, *Consult. Tom.* II., *Cas.* 125.

---

[44] Bleeding piles returned every month.

[45] In consequence of itch driven off by external applications, loss of blood up to eight pounds within a few hours colic, fever, etc.

[46] After the expulsion of itch a most violent colic, pain in the region of the left lower ribs, restlessness, lingering fever, anxiety and obstinate constipation.

[47] A young peasant had driven off the itch with ointment, and shortly after he suffered from suppression of urine, vomiting, and at times from a pain in the left loin. Still he, after a while, passed urine a few times, but only a little, of dark color and attended with pains. In vain the attempt was made to empty it with a catheter. At last the whole body swelled up, difficult and slow respiration ensued, and he died on about the twenty-first day after the supression of the itch. The bladder contained two pounds of urine just as dark, but the abdominal cavity, water, which when held for awhile over the fire thickened into a sort of albumen.

[48] A man rubbed himself with mercurial ointment against the itch, when there followed an erysipelatous inflammation in the neck, of which he died after five weeks.

Ulcers, Unzer *Arzt. Th.* V., St. 301.[49] **Pelargus,** as above, *Jahrg.*, 1723, p. 673.[50] *Breslauer Samm.*, 1727, p. 107.[51] **Muzell,** *Wahrnehm*, II., *Cas.* 6.[52] **Riedlin,** the son, *Cent. obs.* 38.[53] **Alberti-Gorn,** *Diss. de scabi.*, p. 24. Halle, 1718.

Caries, Richard, as above.

Swelling of the Bones of the Knee. Valsalva in **Morgagni,** *de sede et caus. morb.* I. art. 13.

Pain in the Bones, *Hamburger Magaz.*, XVIII., p. 3, 253.

Rachitis and Marasmus in Children, Fr. Hoffman. *Kinderkrankh. Leipz.* 1741, p. 132.

Fever, B. V. Faventinus, *Medicina empir.*, p. 260. **Ramazzini,** *Constit. epid. urbis.* II. No. 32, 1691.[54] **J. C. Carl** in *Act. Nat. Cur.* VI., *obs.* 16.[55]

---

[49] A woman, after using a mercurial ointment against itch, had a putrescent eruption all over her body, so that whole pieces of flesh rotted away; she died in a few days with the greatest pains.

[50] A youth of 16 years had the itch for some time; when this passed away ulcers broke out on the legs

[51] After rubbing with an ointment against the itch there followed with a man of 50 years tearing pains in the left shoulder for five weeks, when several ulcers broke out in the arm-pit.

[52] A quack gave a student an ointment for the itch, from which it disappeared indeed, but instead of it an incurable ulcer broke out in the mouth.

[53] A student who had been for a long time afflicted with the itch drove it off with an ointment, and instead of this there broke out ulcers on his arms and legs, and glandular swellings in the armpits. These ulcers were finally cured by external applications, when he was seized with dyspnœa and then with dropsy, and from these he died.

[54] Many observations are found there, respecting cases where the itch, being driven off by ointments, there followed fever and blackish urine, and where, when the itch was brought back to the skin, the fever disappeared and the urine became like that of a healthy person.

[55] A man and a woman had an eruption of itch on the hand, of many years' standing, and as often as it dried up fever always ensued, and as soon as this came to an end the eruption of itch again returned; and yet this itch extended but to a small part of the body and was not driven off by external applications.

Fever, Reil, *Memorab. Fasc.* III., p. 169.[56] **Pelargus,** as above; Jahrg., 1721, p. 276,[57] and *ibid. Jahrg.*, 1723.[58] **Amatus,** *Lusit. Cent.* II., Cor., 33. **Schiller,** *Diss. de scabie humida*, Erford, 1747, p. 44.[59] **J. J. Fick,** *Exercitatio med. de scabie retropulsa*, Halle, 1710, § 2.[60] **Pelargus,** as above, *Jahrg.*, 1722, p. 122.[61] Also *Jahrg.*, 1723, p. 10, p. 14[62] and p. 291. **C. G. Lud-**

---

[56] Itch was suppressed by a fever that set in; when the fever was removed it returned.

[57] A mother put ointment on the *tinea* of a boy of nine years; it passed away, but there followed a violent fever.

[58] A child, one year old, had had for some time *tinea capitis* and an eruption on the face; both these had shortly before dried up, when there followed heat, cough and diarrhœa. A return of the eruption on the head gave alleviation.

[59] A woman of 43 years, long afflicted with dry itch, rubbed her joints with an ointment of *Sulphur* and *Mercury*, and thus drove it off; this was followed by pains under the right ribs, lassitude in all the limbs, heat and feverish irritation. After using sudorific remedies for six days, large vesicles of itch broke out all over the body.

[60] Two youths, brothers, drove off the itch by one and the same remedy, but they lost all appetite, a dry cough and a lingering fever set in, they became emaciated and fell into a slumbrous stupor, so that they would have died if the eruption had not luckily re-appeared on the skin.

[61] With a three-year-old child when *tinea capitis* had disappeared of itself, there arose a violent fever on the chest, cough and weariness, and it only recovered when the eruption re-appeared on the head.

[62] A journeyman purse-maker, who had to make some embroidery, drove off his frequent itch with *Lead* ointment. Scarcely was the itch drying off in consequence, when he was seized with chills, heat, dyspnœa and a rattling cough, of which he suffocated on the fourth day.

wig, *Advers. med.* II., pp. 157–160.[63] **Morgagni,** as ab., X., *art.* 9;[64] XXI., *art.* 31;[65] XXXVIII., *art.* 22;[66] LV., *art.* 3.[67]

---

[63] A vigorous, healthy man of 30 years was taken with the itch and drove the eruption from the skin, but was then seized with a catarrhal fever with an uncontrollable perspiration; he was slowly recovering from it when he was seized without any further cause by another fever. The attacks began with anxiety and headache, and increased with heat, a quick pulse and morning sweats. There was added an unusual sinking of the strength, and delirious speech, anxious tossing about, a sobbing respiration with suffocation—a disease which despite all medicines ended with death.

[64] With a boy the itch passed away of itself; this was followed by fever. The itch now appeared more violent and the fever passed away, but the child grew thin, and when the itch again dried up there followed diarrhœa, convulsions and soon afterwards death.

[65] Itch disappeared from the skin of itself, on which lingering fever, expectoration of pus and lastly death followed, and at the autopsy the left lungs were found full of pus.

[66] A woman of 30 years had for a long time pain in the limbs and a strong eruption of itch, which she drove off with ointment, when she was attacked by fever with violent heat, thirst and raging headache, which was accompanied with delirious speech, uncontrollable dyspnœa, tumefaction of the body and great distension of the abdomen. She died on the sixth day of the fever. The abdomen contained much air, and especially the stomach was distended with air, filling half of the abdomen.

[67] A man whose *tinea capitis* had passed off from intense cold, was seized after eight days with a malignant fever, with vomiting, accompanied at last with hiccough; he died in consequence on the ninth day.

In the same article **Morgagni** mentions the case of a man who, having scabs from itch on the arms and on other parts, drove off nearly the whole eruption by a sulphurated shirt, but was seized at once with drawing pains on the whole body combined with fever, so that he could neither rest at night nor move about in the daytime; also the tongue and the fauces were thus attacked. With

Fever. **Lanzonus,** in *Eph. Nat. Cur.*, *Dec.* III., *ann.* 9 and 10, *obs.* 16 and 113. **Hoechstetter,** *Obs. med.*, *Dec.* VIII., Cas. 8.[68] **Triller.** **Wehle,** *Diss. nullam medicinam interdum esse optimam*, Witemb., 1754.[69] **Fick,** as ab., § 1.[70] **Waldschmidt,** *Opera.*, p. 241. **Gerbizius,** in *Eph. Nat. Cur.*, *Dec.* III., *ann.* 2, *obs.* 167. **Amatus,** *Lusit.*, Cent. II., Curat. 33.[71] **Fr. Hoffmann,** *Med. rat. system*, T. III., p. 175.[72]

Tertian Intermittent Fever. **Pelargus,** as ab., Jahrg., 1722, p. 103, cfr. with p. 79.[73] **Juncker,** as ab., *tab.* 79;

---

much trouble the eruption was brought out again on the skin, and thus his health was restored.

[68]A malignant fever with opisthotonus from driving off the itch.

[69]A young merchant had driven off the itch with ointment, when he was suddenly seized with such hoarseness that he could not speak a loud word; then followed dry asthma, loathing of food, severe cough, troublesome especially at night and robbing him of sleep; violent, ill-smelling nightsweats, and, despite all medical treatment, death.

[70]A burgomaster, 60 years of age, was infected with the itch, and suffered unspeakably from it through the nights; he used many medicines in vain, and at last was taught by a beggar a so-called infallible remedy, composed of *oleum laurinum*, flowers of sulphur and lard. Having rubbed with this several times he was, indeed, freed from the eruption, but soon after he was seized with a violent chill, followed by an excessive heat all over the body, vehement thirst, a gasping asthma, sleeplessness, violent trembling all over the body and great lassitude, so that on the fourth day he expired.

[71] From the same cause a fever combined with insanity, precipitating death.

[72]After driving off itch, most frequently acute fevers with a great sinking of the strength follow. In one such case the fever lasted seven days, when the eruption of itch re-appeared and stopped the fever.

[73]A boy of 15 years for a long time had *tinea capitis* and had re-

Eph. Nat. Cur. Dec. I., *ann.* 4. **Welsch,** *Obs.* 15. **Sauvages,** *Spec.* 11. **De Hautesierk,** *Obs., Tom.* II., p. 300; *Comment. Lipsienses* XIX., p. 297.

Quartan Fever, Thom. Bartholinus, *Cap.* 4, *hist.* 35. **Sennert,** *Paralip.*, p. 116. **Fr. Hoffman,** *Med. rat. system* III., p. 175.[74]

Vertigo and a Total Sinking of the Strength, Gabelchofer, *Obs. Med. Cent.* II., *obs.* 42.

Vertigo Like Epilepsy, Fr. Hoffmann, *Consult. Med.* I., *Cas.* 12.[75]

Epilepsy Like Vertigo, Fr. Hoffmann, as ab., p. 30.[76]

---

ceived from *Pelargus* a strong purgative to cure it; he was seized with pain in the back, cutting pains during micturition, followed by tertian fever.

[74] Old people have especially dry itch, and if this is driven off by external applications, usually quartan fever ensues, which vanishes as soon as the itch re-appears on the skin.

[75] A count, 57 years old, had suffered for three years with dry itch. It was driven off, and he enjoyed for two years an apparently good health, only he had during this time two attacks of vertigo, which gradually so increased that once after finishing his meal he was seized with such vertigo that he would have fallen to the floor if he had not been supported. He was covered with an icy perspiration, his limbs trembled, all the parts of his body were as dead, and he repeatedly vomited up a sour substance. A similar attack followed six weeks later, then once a month for three months. He indeed retained consciousness, but there always followed heaviness of the head and a drunken stupor. At last these attacks came daily, though in a milder form. He could not read, nor think, nor turn around quickly, nor stoop down. This was attended with sadness, sorrowful, anxious thoughts and sighs.

[76] A woman of 36 years had the itch driven from the skin a few years before with mercurial remedies. Her menses became irregular, and were often interrupted for ten or even fifteen weeks; she was at the same time constipated. Four years ago during preg-

Convulsions, Juncker, as ab. tab., 53. **Hoechstetter,** *Eph. Nat. Cur. Dec.* 8, *Cas.* 3. *Eph. nat. cur. dec.* 2, *ann. obs.* 35, and *ann.* 5, *obs.* 224. **D. W. Triller. Welle,** *Diss. nullam medicinam interdum esse optimam,* Viteb., 1754, § 13, 14.[77] **Sicelius,** *Decas Casuum* I., *Cas.* 5.[78] **Pelargus,** as ab., *Jahrg.*, 1723, p. 545.[79]

---

nancy she was seized with vertigo, and she would suddenly fall down while standing or walking. While sitting she would retain her senses during the vertigo and could speak, eat and drink. At her first attack she felt in her left foot, as it were, a crawling sensation and formication, which terminated in a violent jerking up and down of the feet. In time these attacks took away consciousness, and afterwards, in traveling in a carriage, there came an attack of real epilepsy, which returned thrice in the following winter. During these attacks she could not speak; she did not, indeed, turn her thumbs inward, but yet there was foam at her mouth. The sensation of formication in the left foot announced the attack, and when this sensation reached the pit of the stomach it suddenly brought on the fit. This epilepsy was removed by a woman with five powders, but instead of it her vertigo re-appeared, but much more violently than before. It also commenced with a crawling sensation in the left foot, which rose up to the heart; this was attended with great anxiety and fear, as if she were falling down from a height. and while supposing that she had fallen she lost consciousness and speech; at the same time her limbs moved convulsively. But, also, outside of these attacks the least touch of her feet caused her the most intense pain, as if from a boil. This was attended with severe pains and heat in the head and with loss of memory.

[77]After an itch driven away by ointment there followed, with a girl, a most profound swoon, and soon after the most terrible convulsions and death.

[78]A girl of 17, in consequence of *tinea capitis* which disappeared of itself, was seized with continual heat in the head and attacks of headache. She sometimes suddenly started up as if from fright, and while awake she was seized with convulsive motions of the limbs, especially of the arms and hands, as also with oppression in the pit of the stomach, as if her breast was laced together, with moaning; then her limbs would jerk convulsively and she would start up.

[79]A full-grown man who had been for some time affected with tremor of the hands had his *tinea* dry up. He was thereupon seized with great lassitude and red patches, without heat, broke out on his body. The tremor passed over into convulsive shaking,

Epileptic Convulsions and

Epilepsy, J. C. Carl in *Act. Nat. Cur.* VI., obs. 16.[80] **E. Hagendorn,** as above, *hist.* 9.[81] **Fr. Hoffmann,** *Consult. med.* I., *Cas.* 31;[82] *ibid. med. rat. syst. T.* IV., P. III., *Cap.* I., and in *Kinderkrankheiten*, p. 108. **Sauvages,** *Nosol. spec.* 11. **De Hautesierk,** *obs. T.* II., p. 300. **Sennert,** *prax.* III., *Cap.* 44. *Eph. Nat. Cur. Dec.* III., *ann.* 2, *obs.* 29. **Gruling,** *obs. Med. Cent.* III., *obs.* 73. **Th. Bartolin,** *Cent.* III., *hist.* 20. **Fabr. de Hilden,** *Cent.* III., *obs.* 10.[83] **Riedlin,** *lin. med. ann.*, 1696, *Maj. obs.* 1.[84] **Lentilius,** *Miscell. med. pr.*, P. I., p. 32. **G. W. Wedel,** *Diss. de aegro epileptico, Jen.*, 1673.[85] **Herrm. Grube,** *de arcanis medicorum non arcanis, Hafn.*, 1673,

---

bloody matter was discharged from his nose and his ears, he also coughed up blood, and he died on 23d day amidst convulsions.

[80]A man who had driven off a frequently occurring eruption of itch with an ointment fell into epileptic convulsions, which disappeared again when the eruption re-appeared on the skin.

[81]A youth of 18 years drove off the itch with a mercurial ointment and two months after he was unexpectedly seized with convulsions, which attacked all the limbs of the body, now this, now that, with painful constriction of the breast and the neck, coldness of the limbs and great weakness. The fourth day he was seized with epilepsy, foaming at the mouth, while the limbs were strangely contorted. The epilepsy only yielded when the eruption returned.

[82]With a boy, whose tinea had been driven off by rubbing it with almond oil.

[83]With children, combined with suffocating catarrh.

[84]A servant girl after twice rubbing her itch with ointment had an attack of epilepsy.

[85]A youth of 18, who had driven out itch with mercurial remedies, was seized a few weeks later with epilepsy, which returned after four weeks with the new moon.

p. 165.[86] **Tulpius,** *obs. lib.* I., *Cap.* 8.[87] **Th. Thompson,** *Medic. Rathpflege, Leipzig*, 1779, pp. 107, 108.[88] **Hundertmark,** as ab., p. 32.[89] **Fr. Hoffmann,** *Consult. med.* I., Cas. 28, p. 141.[90]

---

[86]A boy of 7 months was seized with epilepsy, while the parents were unwilling to acknowledge that he had had the itch. But when the physician enquired more particularly the mother confessed that the little boy had some vesicles of itch on the sole of the foot, which had soon yielded to lead ointment; the child, as she said, had no other sign of the itch. The physician correctly recognized in this the only cause of the epilepsy.

[87]Two children were freed from epilepsy by the breaking out of humid tinea, but the epilepsy returned when the tinea was incautiously driven off.

[88]Five-year-old itch passed away, and this, after several years, produced epilepsy.

[89]The itch in a youth of 20 years was suppressed by a purgative, which was allowed to act violently for several days, after which he for two years suffered the most violent convulsions, until, through the use of birch-juice, the itch was brought back to the skin.

[90]A young man of 17 years, of vigorous constitution and good intelligence, was attacked three years ago, after itch had been driven out, first by hemoptysis and then by epilepsy, which grew worse through medicines until the fits came on every two hours. Another surgeon, through frequent blood-lettings and many medicines, effected that he remained free from epilepsy for four weeks, but soon afterwards the epilepsy returned while he was taking his noon-day nap, and the patient had two or three fits in the night; at the same time he was attacked with a very severe cough and suffocating catarrh, especially during the nights, when he expectorated a very fetid fluid. He was confined to his bed. At last, after much medicine, the disease increased so much that he had ten fits at night and eight during the day. Nevertheless he never in these fits either clenched his hands or had foam at his mouth. His memory is weakened. The attacks come at the approach of meal-time, but more frequently after meals. During his nightly attacks he remains in the deepest sleep without awaking, but in

Apoplexy. **Cummius** in *Eph. Nat. Cur. Dec.* I., *ann.* 1, *obs.* 58. **Mobius,** *Institut. med.*, p. 65. **J. J. Wepfer,** *Histor. Apoplect. Amstel.*, 1724, p. 457.

Paralysis, Hoechstetter, *Obs. med. Dec.* VIII., *obs.* 8, p. 245. *Journal de Méd.*, 1760, Sept., p. 211. **Unzer** *Arzt* VI., *St.* 301.[91] **Hundertmark,** as above, p. 33.[92] **Krause. Schubert,** *Diss. de scabie humani corp., Lips.*, 1779, p. 23.[93] **Karl Wenzel,** as above, p. 174.

Melancholy, Reil, *Memorab. Fasc.*, III., p. 177.[94]

Insanity, Landais in **Roux,** *Journ. de Médicine*, Tom. 41. **Amat. Lusitanus,** *Curat. med. Cent.* II., *Cur.* 74. **J. H. Schulze, Brune,** *Diss. Casus aliquot mente alienatorum*, Halle, 1707. Cas. 1, p. 5.[95] **F. H. Waitz,** *medic.-chirurg*

---

the morning he feels as if bruised all over. The only warning of a fit consists in his rubbing his nose and drawing up his left foot, but then he suddenly falls down.

[91]A woman, after having the itch driven out, had paralysis of one leg and remained lame.

[92]After driving off the itch with sulphur ointment, a man of 53 years had hemiplegia.

[93]A minister, who for a long time had in vain used internal remedies against the itch, finally grew tired of it and drove it off with ointment, when his upper extremities were, in a measure, paralyzed and a hard, thick skin formed in the palms of the hands, full of bloody chaps and insufferable itching.

In the same place the author mentions also a woman whose fingers contracted from an itch driven out by external means; she suffered from them a long time.

[94]He found an idiotic melancholy arise in consequence of suppressed itch; when the itch broke out again the melancholy disappeared.

[95]A student, 20 years old, had the humid itch, which so covered his hands that he became incapable of attending to his work. It was driven off by sulphur ointment. But shortly after it appeared how much his health had suffered from it. He became insane,

Aufsätze, *Th.* 1, p. 130.[96] *Altenburg*, 1791. **Richter** in *Hufel. Journal*, XV., II. **Grossmann** in **Baldinger's** *neuem Magaz.*, XI., I.[97]

Who, after meditating on even these few examples which might be much increased from the writings of the physicians of that time and from my experience,* would remain so thoughtless as to ignore the

---

sang or laughed where it was unbecoming, and ran until he sank to the ground from exhaustion. From day to day he became more sick in soul and body, until at last hemiplegia came on and he died. The intestines were found grown together into a firm mass, studded with little ulcers full of protuberances, some of the size of walnuts, which were filled with a substance resembling gypsum.

[96] The same story.

[97] A man of 50 years with whom, after driving away the itch by ointments, general dropsy had set in; when the itch re-appeared and drove away the swelling, he drove it away again, when he fell into raving madness, while head and neck swelled up to suffocation; at last blindness and complete suppression of urine were added. Artificial irritants applied to the skin and a strong emetic brought back the itch again; when the eruption extended over the whole body all the former accidents disappeared.

*An opponent, of the old school, has reproached me that I have not adduced my own experience to prove that the chronic maladies, when they are not of syphilitic or sycotic origin, spring from the miasma of itch, as such proofs from experience would have been convincing. Oho! If the examples here adduced by me from both the older and from modern non-Homœopathic writings have not yet enough convincing proof, I should like to know what other examples (even my own not excepted) could be conceived of as more striking proofs? How often (and I might say almost always) have opponents of the old school refused all credence to the observations of honorable Homœopathic physicians, because they were not made before their own eyes and because the names of the patients were only indicated with a letter; as if private patients would allow their names to be used! Why should I endure the like? And do I not prove my point in a manner most indubitable and most free from partisanship through the experience of so many other honest practitioners?

great evil hidden within, the *Psora*, of which evil the eruption of itch and its other forms, the *tinea capitis*, milk crust, tetter, etc., are only indications announcing the internal, monstrous disease of the whole organism, only local external symptoms which act vicariously and mitigatingly for the internal disease? Who, after reading even the few cases described, would hesitate to acknowledge that the *Psora*, as already stated, is the *most destructive* of all chronic miasmas? Who would be so stolid as to declare, with the later allopathic physicians, that the itch-eruption, tinea and tetters are only situated superficially upon the skin and may, therefore, without fear, be driven out through external means since the internal of the body has no part in it and retains its health?

Surely, among all the crimes which the modern physicians of the old school are guilty of, this is the most hurtful, shameful and unpardonable!

The man who, from the examples given and from innumerable others of a like nature, is not willing to see the exact opposite of that assertion blinds himself on purpose and works intentionally for the destruction of mankind.

Or are they so little instructed as to the nature of all the miasmatic maladies connected with diseases of the skin that they do not know that they all take a similar course in their origin? And that all such miasmas become first internal maladies of the whole system before their external assuaging symptoms appear on the skin?

We shall more closely elucidate this process, and in consequence we shall see that all miasmatic maladies which show peculiar local ailments on the skin are always present as internal maladies in the system *before* they show their local symptoms externally upon the skin; but that only in acute diseases, after taking their course through a certain number of days, the local symptom, together with the internal disease, is wont to disappear, which then leaves the body free from both. In chronic miasmas, however, the outer local symptoms may either be driven from the skin or may disappear of itself, while the internal disease, if uncured, neither wholly nor in part ever leaves the system; on the contrary, it continually increases with the years, unless healed by art.

I must here dwell the more circumstantially on this process of nature, because the common physicians, especially of modern days, are so deficient in vision; or, more correctly stated, so blind that although they could, as it were, handle and feel this process in the origin and development of acute miasmatic eruptional diseases, they nevertheless neither surmised nor observed the like process in chronic diseases, and therefore declared their local symptoms as secondary growths and impurities existing merely externally on the skin, without any internal fundamental disease, and this as well with the chancre and the fig-wart as with the eruption of itch, and, therefore—since they overlooked the chief disease or perhaps even boldly denied it—by a mere external treatment and destruction of these local ailments they have brought unspeakable misfortunes on suffering humanity.

With respect to the origin of these three chronic maladies, as in the acute, miasmatic eruptional diseases, three different important moments are to be more attentively considered than has hitherto been done: *First*, the time of infection; *secondly*, the period of time during which the whole organism is being penetrated by the disease infused, until it has developed within; and *thirdly*, the breaking out of the external ailment, whereby nature externally demonstrates the completion of the internal development of the miasmatic malady throughout the whole organism.

The infection with miasmas, as well of the acute as of the above mentioned chronic diseases, takes place, without doubt, in *one single moment*, and that moment, the one most favorable for infection.

When the small-pox or the cow-pox catches, this happens in the moment when in vaccination the morbid fluid in the bloody scratch of the skin comes in contact with the exposed nerve, which then, irrevocably, dynamically communicates the disease to the vital force (to the whole nervous system) in the same moment. After this moment of infection no ablution, cauterizing or burning, not even the cutting off of the part which has caught and received the infection, can again destroy or undo the development of the disease within. Small-pox, cow-pox, measles, etc., nevertheless will complete their course within, and the fever peculiar to each will break out with its small-pox, cow-pox, measles,* etc., *after a few days*, when the internal disease has developed and completed itself.

* We may justly ask: Is there in any probability any miasma in the world, which, when it has infected from without, does not first make the whole organism sick before the signs of it externally manifest themselves? We can only answer this question with, *no*, there is none!

The same is the case, not to mention several other acute miasmas, also when the skin of man is contaminated with the blood of cattle affected with anthrax. If, as is frequently the case, the anthrax has infected and caught on, all ablutions of the skin are in vain; the black or gangrenous blister, nearly always fatal, nevertheless, always comes out after four or five days (usually in the affected spot); *i. e.*, as soon as the whole living organism has transformed itself to this terrible disease.

(It is just so with the infection of half-acute miasmas without eruption. Among many persons bitten by mad dogs—thanks to the benign ruler of the world—only few are infected, rarely the twelfth; often, as I

Does it not take three, four or five days after vaccination is effected, before the vaccinated spot becomes inflamed? Does not the sort of fever developed—the sign of the completion of the disease—appear even later, when the protecting pock has been fully formed; *i. e.*, on the seventh or eighth day?

Does it not take ten to twelve days after infection with small-pox, before the inflammatory fever and the outbreak of the small-pox on the skin take place?

What has nature been doing with the infection received in these ten or twelve days? Was it not necessary to first embody the disease in the whole organism before nature was enabled to kindle the fever, and to bring out the eruption on the skin?

Measles also require ten or twelve days after infection or inoculation before this eruption with its fever appears. After infection with scarlet fever seven days usually pass before the scarlet fever, with the redness of the skin, breaks out.

What then did nature do with the received miasma during the intervening days? What else but to incorporate the whole disease of measles or scarlet fever in the entire living organism before she had completed the work, so as to be enabled to produce the measles and the scarlet fever with their eruption.

myself have observed, only one out of twenty or thirty persons bitten. The others, even if ever so badly mangled by the mad dog, usually all recover, even if they are not treated by a physician or surgeon.*) But with whomsoever the poison acts, it has taken effect in the moment when the person was bitten, and the poison has then communicated itself to the nearest nerves and, therefore, without contradiction, to the whole system of the nerves, and as soon as the malady has been developed in the whole organism (for this development and completion of the disease nature requires at least several days, often many weeks), the madness breaks out as an acute, quickly fatal disease. Now if the venomous spittle of the mad dog has really taken effect, the infection usually has taken place irrevocably in the moment of contagion, for experience shows that even the immediate excision† and amputation of the infected part does not protect from the progression of the disease within, nor from the breaking out of the hydrophobia—therefore. also, the many

---

* We are indebted especially to the careful English and American physicians for these comforting experiences—to HUNTER and HOULSTON (in *London Med. Journal*, Vol. I.), and to VAUGHAN, SHADWELL and PERCIVAL, whose observations are recorded in Jam. Mease's "*On the Hydrophobia, Philadelphia*, 1793."

† An eight-year-old girl, in Glasgow, was bitten by a mad dog on the 21st of March, 1792. A surgeon *immediately exsected the wound altogether*, kept it suppurating and gave Mercury until it produced a mild salivation, which was kept up for two weeks; nevertheless hydrophobia broke out on the 27th of April and the patient died on the 29th of April. M. DUNCAN'S *Med. Comment, Dec.* II., *Vol.* VII., *Edinb.*, 1793, and *The New London Med. Journ.*, II.

hundreds of other much lauded external means for cleansing, cauterizing and suppurating the wound of the bite can protect just as little from the breaking out of the hydrophobia.

From the progress of all these miasmatic diseases we may plainly see that, after the contagion from without, the malady connected with it in the interiors of the whole man must first be developed; *i. e.*, the whole interior man must first have become thoroughly sick of small-pox, measles or scarlet fever, before these various eruptions can appear on the skin.

For all these *acute* miasmatic diseases the human constitution possesses that process, which, as a rule, is so beneficent: to wipe them out (*i. e.*, the specific fever together with the specific eruption) in the course of from two to three weeks, and of itself to extinguish them again, through a kind of decision (*crisis*), from the organism, so that man then is wont to be entirely healed of them and, indeed, in a short time, unless he be killed by them.*

---

*Or have these various, acute, half-spiritual miasms the peculiar characteristic that—after they have penetrated the vital force in the first moment of the contagion (and each one in its own way has produced disease) and then, like parasites, have quickly grown up within it and have usually developed themselves by their peculiar fever after producing their fruit (the mature cutaneous eruption which is again capable of producing its miasma)—they again die out and leave the living organism again free to recover?

On the other hand, are not the chronic miasmas disease-parasites, which continue to live as long as the man seized by them is alive, and which have their fruit in the eruption originally produced by them (the itch-pustule, the chancre and the fig-wart, which in turn are capable of infecting others), and which do not die off of themselves like the acute miasmas, but can only be exterminated and

In the chronic miasmatic diseases nature observes *the same course* with respect to the mode of contagion and the antecedent formation of the internal disease, before the external declarative symptoms of its internal completion manifests itself on the surface of the body, but then that great remarkable difference from the acute diseases shows itself, that in the chronic miasmata the entire internal disease, as we have mentioned before, remains in the organism during the whole life, yea, it increases with every year, if it is not exterminated and thoroughly cured *by art.*

Of these chronic miasmata I shall for this purpose only adduce those two which we know somewhat more exactly, namely, the *venereal chancre* and the *itch.*

In impure coition there arises, most probably at the very moment in the spot which is touched and rubbed, the specific contagion.

If this contagion has taken effect, then the whole living body is in consequence seized with it. Immediately after the moment of contagion the formation of the venereal disease in the whole of the interior begins.

In that part of the sexual organs where the infection has taken place nothing unnatural is noticed in the first days, nothing diseased, inflamed or corroded; *so also all washing and cleansing of the parts immediately after the impure coition is in vain.* The spot remains healthy according to appearance, only the internal organism is called into activity by the infection (which

---

annihilated by a *counter-infection*, by means of the potency of a medicinal disease quite similar to it and stronger than it (the antipsoric), so that the patient is delivered from them and recovers his health?

occurs usually in a moment), so as to incorporate the venereal miasma and to become thoroughly diseased with the venereal malady.

Only when this penetration of all the organs by the disease caught has been effected, only when the whole being has been changed into a man entirely venereal, *i. e.*, when the development of the venereal disease has been completed, only then diseased nature endeavors to mitigate the internal evil and to soothe it by producing a local symptom, which first shows itself as a vesicle (usually in the spot originally infected), and later breaks out into a painful ulcer called the chancre; this does not appear before five, seven or fourteen days, sometimes, though rarely, not before three, four or five weeks after the infection. This is, therefore, manifestly a chancre ulcer, which acts vicariously for the internal malady, and which has been produced from within by the organism after it has become venereal through and through, and is able through its touch to communicate also to other men the same miasma, *i. e.*, the venereal disease.

Now, if the entire disease thus arising is again extinguished through the internally given specific remedy, then the chancre also is healed and the man recovers.

But if the chancre is destroyed through local applitions* before the internal disease is healed—and this is

---

*The venereal disease not only breaks out through the removal of the chancre by the cautery—in which case some wretched casuists have considered syphilis as resulting from the driving back of the poison out of the chancre into the interior of the body, which up to this time is supposed by them to have been healthy—no, even after the quick removal of the chancre without any external stimu-

still a daily practice with physicians of the old school —the miasmatic, chronic, venereal disease remains in the organism as syphilis, and it is aggravated, if not then cured internally, from year to year until the end of man's life, even the most robust constitution being unable to annihilate it within itself.

Only through the cure of the venereal disease, which pervades the whole internal of the body (as I have taught and practiced for many years), the chancre, its local symptom, will also simultaneously be cured in the most effective manner, and this is best affected without the use of any external application for its removal— while the merely local destruction of the chancre, without any previous general cure and deliverance of man from the internal disease, is followed by the most certain outbreak of syphilis with its sufferings.

Psora (itch disease), like *syphilis*, is a miasmatic chronic disease, and its original development is similar.

The itch disease is, however, also the *most contagious* of all chronic miasmata, far more infectious than the other two chronic miasmata, the venereal chancre disease and the figwart disease. To effect the infection with the latter there is required a certain amount of friction in the most tender parts of the body, which

lants, the venereal disease breaks out, which gives additional confirmation, if this were needed, of the indubitable pre-existence of syphilis in the system. "*Petit* cut off a part of the *labia minora*, in which for some days a venereal chancre had appeared; the wound healed, indeed, but the venereal disease broke out notwithstanding." M. s. *Fabre, Lettres, supplément à son traité des maladies vénériennes, Paris*, 1786. Of course! because the venereal disease was present in the whole interior of the body even before the outbreak of the chancre.

are the most rich in nerves and covered with the thinnest cuticle, as in the genital organs, unless the miasma should touch a wounded spot. But *the miasma of the itch needs only to touch the general skin*, especially with tender children. The disposition of being affected with the miasma of the itch is found with almost everyone and under almost all circumstances, which is not the case with the other two miasmata.

No other chronic miasma infects more generally, more surely, more easily and more absolutely than the miasma of itch; as already stated, it is the most contagious of all. It is communicated so easily that even the physician, hurrying from one patient to another, in feeling the pulse has unconsciously* inoculated other patients with it; wash which is washed with wash infected with the itch;† new gloves, which had been tried on by an itch patient; a strange lodging place, a strange towel used for drying oneself have communicated this tinder of contagion; yea, often a babe, when being born, is infected while passing through the organs of the mother, who may be infected (as is not infrequently the case) with this disease; or the babe receives this unlucky infection through the hand of the midwife, which has been infected by another parturient woman (or previously); or, again, a suckling may be infected by its nurse, or, while on her arm, by her caresses or the caresses of a strange person with unclean hands, not to mention the thousands of other possible ways in which things polluted with this invisi-

---

* CAR. MUSITANI, *Opera de tumoribus*, *Cap.* 20.

† As WILLIS has noticed in TURNER, *des maladies de la peau, traduit de l'anglois, à Paris*, 1783, *Tom.* II , *Cap.* 3, p. 77.

ble miasma may touch a man in the course of his life, and which often can in no way be anticipated or guarded against, so that men who have never been infected by the *Psora* are the exception. We need not to hunt for the causes of infection in crowded hospitals, factories, prisons, or in orphan houses, or in the filthy huts of paupers; even in active life, in retirement, and in the rich classes, the itch creeps in. The hermit on Montserrat escapes it as rarely in his rocky cell as the little prince in his swaddling clothes of cambric.

As soon as the miasma of itch, *e. g.*, touches the hand, in the moment when it has taken effect, it no more remains local. Henceforth all washing and cleansing of the spot avail nothing. Nothing is seen on the skin during the first days; it remains unchanged, and, according to appearance, healthy. There is no eruption or itching to be noticed on the body during these days, not even on the spot infected. The nerve which was first affected by the miasma has already communicated it in an invisible dynamic manner to the nerves of the rest of the body, and the living organism has at once, all unperceived, been so penetrated by this specific excitation that it has been compelled to appropriate this miasma gradually to itself until the change of the whole being to a man thoroughly psoric, and thus the internal development of the *Psora*, has reached completion.

Only when the whole organism feels itself transformed by this peculiar chronic-miasmatic disease, the diseased vital force endeavors to alleviate and to soothe the internal malady through the establishment of a suitable local symptom on the skin, the itch-vesicles. So long as this eruption continues in its normal form the internal *Psora*, with its secondary ailments, cannot break forth, but must remain covered, slumbering, latent and bound.

Usually it takes six, seven or ten, perhaps even fourteen days from the moment of infection before the transformation of the entire internal organism into *Psora* has been effected. Then only there follows after a slight or more severe chill in the evening and a general heat, followed by perspiration in the following night (a little fever which by many persons is ascribed to a cold and therefore disregarded), the outbreak of the vesicles of itch, at first fine, as if from miliary fever, but afterwards enlarging on the skin*—first in the region of the spot first infected, and, indeed, accompanied with a *voluptuously tickling itching*, which may be called *unbearably agreeable* (*Grimmen*), which compels the patient so irresistibly to rub and to scratch the vesicles of itch, that, if a person restrains himself forcibly from rubbing or scratching, a shudder passes over the skin of the whole body. This *rubbing* and *scratching*, indeed, satisfies somewhat for a few moments, but there then *follows immediately a long-continued burning of the part affected.* Late in the evening and before midnight this itching is most frequent and most unbearable.

---

*Far from being an independent, merely local, cutaneous disease, the vesicles or pustules of itch are the reliable proof that the completion of the internal *Psora* has already been effected, and the eruption is merely an integrating factor of the same, for this peculiar eruption and this peculiar itching make a part of the essence of the whole disease in its natural, least dangerous state.

The vesicles of itch contain in the first hours of their formation a lymph clear as water, but this quickly changes into pus, which fills the tip of the vesicle.

The itching not only compels the patient to rub, but on account of its violence, as before mentioned, to rub and scratch open the vesicles; and the humor pressed out furnishes abundant material for infecting the surroundings of the patient and also other persons not yet infected. The extremities defiled even to an imperceptible degree with this lymph, so also the wash, the clothes and the utensils of all kinds, when touched, propagate the disease.

Only this skin symptom of the *Psora* which has permeated the whole organism (and which is more manifestly falling under the cognizance of the senses has the name of *itch*), only this eruption, as well as the sores which later arise from it and are attended on their borders with the itching peculiar to *Psora*, as also the herpes which has this peculiar itching and which becomes humid when rubbed (the tetter), as also the *tinea capitis*—these alone can propagate this disease to other persons, because they alone contain the communicable miasma of the *Psora*. But the remaining secondary symptoms of the *Psora*, which in time manifest themselves after the disappearance or the artificial expulsion of the eruption, *i. e.*, the general *Psoric* ailments, cannot at all communicate this disease to others. They are, so far as we know, just as little able to transfer the *Psora* to others, as the secondary symptoms of the venereal disease are able to infect other men (as first observed and taught by J. HUNTER) with syphilis.

When the itch-eruption has only lately broken out and is not yet widely spread on the skin, nothing of the general internal malady of the *Psora* is as yet to be noticed in the state of the patient. The eruptional symptom acts as a substitute for the internal malady and keeps the *Psora* with its secondary ailments as it were latent and confined.*

In this state, the disease is most easily cured through specific remedies internally administered.

But if the disease is allowed to advance in its peculiar course without the use of an internal curative remedy or an external application to drive away the eruption, the whole disease within *rapidly* increases, and this increase of the internal malady makes necessary a corresponding increase of the skin symptom. The itch-eruption, therefore, in order to be able to soothe and to keep latent the increased internal malady, has to spread and must finally cover the whole surface of the body.

Yet even at this acme of the disease the patient still appears healthy in every other respect; all the symptoms of the internal *Psora*, now so much increased, still remain covered and assuaged through the skin-symptom augmented in the same proportion. But so

---

* As also the chancre, when not expelled, acts vicariously and soothingly for the syphilis within, and does not permit the venereal disease to break out, so long as it remains undisturbed in its place. I examined a woman who was free from all the secondary symptoms of the venereal disease; with her a chancre had remained in its place untreated for two years, and had gradually acquired the size of almost an inch in diameter. The best preparation of *Mercury*, internally administered, soon and entirely healed, not only the internal malady, but also the chancre.

great a torture, as is caused by so unbearable an itching spread over the whole body, even the most robust man cannot continue to bear. He endeavors to free himself from these torments at any price, and, as there is no thorough help for him with the physicians of the old school, he endeavors to secure deliverance at least from this eruption, which itches so unbearably, even if it should cost his life; and the means are soon furnished him, either by other ignorant persons, or by Allopathic physicians and surgeons. He asks deliverance from his external tortures, without suspecting the greater misfortune which unavoidably follows, and is bound to follow, on the expulsion of the external skin-symptoms (which hitherto has acted vicariously for the internal enlarged *Psora*-disease), as has been sufficiently proved by the observations mentioned before. But when he thus drives away such an eruption of itch by external applications, he exposes himself to a similar misfortune, and acts just as unreasonably, as a person who in order to be quickly delivered from poverty, and thus as he supposes to make himself happy, steals a great sum of money, and is, therefore, sent to the dungeon and the gallows.

The longer the itch-disease has already lasted, whether the eruption, as is usually the case, has spread over the greater part of the skin, or whether, owing to a peculiar lack of activity in the skin (as in some cases) the eruption has been confined to a few vesicles of itch*—in both cases, supposing only that the *Psora* together with its skin-symptom has grown old, the ex-

*See the observation to No. 86, p. 67.

pulsion of the eruption of itch, whether greater or smaller or even as small as you please, is attended with the most destructive consequences on account of the internal itch-disease (*Psora*) with its unspeakable sufferings, which, through its long continuance, has increased to a high degree and then unavoidably breaks forth.

But the ignorance of the uninstructed layman may be pardoned if he drives out the itch-eruption and the troublesome itching by a cold shower bath, by rolling in snow, by cupping, or by rubbing the whole skin, or only the skin around the joints, with Sulphur mixed with lard; for he does not know to what dangerous accidents and outbreaks of the *Psora* disease, that lurks within, he thereby opens the door and ingress. But who will pardon the men whose office and duty it is to know the extent of the inevitably following, illimitable misfortune, resulting from the external expulsion of the itch-eruption, owing to the *Psora* which is then aroused from the whole organism, and who ought to have guarded against it in every way by a thorough internal cure of the whole of this disease,* when we

* For even when the itch-disease has reached this high degree, the eruption, together with the internal malady, in one word, the whole *Psora*, may still be healed by the internal, specific homœopathic remedies, with greater difficulty, indeed, than in the beginning, immediately after its origin, but still *far more easily and certainly* than after a complete expulsion of the eruption by mere external applications, when we must cure the internal *Psora* as it brings forth its secondary symptoms and develops into nameless chronic diseases. The itch-disease, though it may have advanced so far, may, nevertheless, in its *entire* state be most easily, certainly and thoroughly cured, together with its external eruption,

see them treat the itch patients all in the same erroneous manner; yea, with even more violent internal and external remedies, with sharp purgatives, with

---

through the suitable internal remedies, without the least local application, just as the venereal chancre disease may *most surely and easily* be thoroughly cured often by the least, single dose of the best preparation of Mercury internally administered--when the chancre, without calling in the aid of the least external remedy, quickly becomes a mild ulcer, and in a few days heals of itself, so that no trace of secondary symptoms (venereal disease) then ever appears or can appear, since the internal symptom has been cured together with the local symptom, as I have taught for many years orally and in my writings, and have proved by my cures of this kind.

How can we excuse the whole host of physicians, who, hitherto, after treating this generally spread venereal disease for more than three hundred years, nevertheless remain so ignorant in recognizing its nature, that in looking at a chancre they even to this day acknowledge nothing diseased in the infected patient, but this same chancre, and do not see the syphilis, which was already present within and had been developed in the whole organism, even before the breaking out of the chancre; and so they blindly suppose, that the chancre is the only venereal evil which is to be extirpated, and that this needs but to be destroyed by external applications, in order to be able to declare the man cured; and this without being instructed, by the many thousand cases in their experience, that by the local extermination of the chancre they have never done anything but injury, as they have only deprived the syphilis pre-existing within of its diverting local symptom, and have thereby compelled the internal malady to break out only the more certainly and dreadfully (and in a manner more difficult to cure), as venereal disease? How can such a universal, pernicious obliquity of vision be excused?

Or why did these physicians never reflect on the origin of the fig-warts? Why did they always overlook the internal universal malady, which is the cause of these excrescences? It is only when this is recognized, that it can be thoroughly cured by its

the Jasser ointment, with lotions of acetate of Lead, with the sublimate of Mercury or sulphate of Zinc, but especially with anointment prepared of fat with flowers

---

homœopathic remedies, which then cause the fig-warts to be healed, without the application of any external means of destruction.

But even if a shadow of an excuse might be offered for this sad negligence and ignorance, and if anyone would claim that these physicians have only had three and one-half centuries, in which to discern clearly the true nature of *syphilis*, and that they might have learned this truth after a still more extended practice (still I have endeavored, though in vain, to convince them of their error a number of years ago and since then from time to time), nevertheless, that general negligence of previous physicians and, I may well say, their obstinate *blindness*, are quite without excuse, in that they did not recognize the internal pre-existing malady, the *Psora*, which lies at the bottom of the itch-disease, which has infected men for several thousands of years, and that they ignored in their proud levity all the facts which point to it, so that they might continue the delusion and leave the world in its destructive infatuation that: *the unbearably itching pustules are only a mere superficial ailment of the skin, and by their local destruction man is delivered form the whole disease, and has fully recovered.*

Not perchance mere medical scribblers, no, the greatest and most celebrated physicians of modern and most modern days have made themselves guilty of this grievous error (or shall I say of this intentional crime), from VON HELMONT even to the latest advocates of the Allopathic medical practice.

By the use of the above-mentioned remedies, they, indeed, usually reached their aim; *i. e.*, the driving away of the eruption and of the itching from the skin, and they supposed in the intoxication of their spirit (or at least they pretended), they had destroyed the disease itself and, indeed, totally, and they sent away the patients, thus abused, assuring them that they were again healthy.

All the sufferings, which follow the one-sided destruction of the cutaneous eruption, which belongs to the natural form of the *Psora*,

of Sulphur or with a preparation of Mercury; with which they lightly and carelessly destroy the eruption, declaring "this is merely an impurity located in the skin, and must be driven out; then everything will be well and the man will be healthy and free from every ailment." Who can pardon them if they are not willing to learn from the many warning examples recorded by the older, more conscientious observers, nor by the many thousands of other examples, which frequently, yea, almost daily, come before their eyes? Yet they cannot see nor be convinced as to the certain, quickly fatal or life-long insidious misfortune they bring upon the itch-patient through the destruction of his eruption, as they thus merely unfetter the internal malady (*Psora*), which is laden with innumerable ailments. This disease is neither destroyed nor cured; and so this thousand-headed monster, instead of being conquered, is inexorably let loose against the deceived patient to his destruction, by tearing down the barriers that shut it in.

It may easily be imagined, as experience also teaches, that the more months a neglected itch-erup-

---

they passed off as a newly arisen disease, owing to quite another origin. In their narrowness of mind, they never regarded the innumerable, plain testimonies of honest observers of earlier days, which record the sad consequences of the local expulsion of the itch-eruption, which often followed so closely, that a man would have to deny his reason, or else acknowledge them as the immediate result of the indwelling severe malady (the *Psora*), which had been deprived of the local symptom (the cutaneous eruption), destined by nature to alleviate the internal malady, whence the uncured internal disease has been compelled to a manifest outbreak of its secondary symptoms.

tion has flourished on the skin, the more surely has internal *Psora*, which underlies it, been able to reach, in even a moderate space of time, a great—and finally its greatest—degree, which dreadful increase it also then proves through the more dangerous consequences, which the expulsion of so inveterate an eruption unavoidably draws after it in every case.

On the other hand, it is just as certain that the eruption of a few vesicles of itch which has broken out only a few days before, in consequence of a recent infection, may be expelled with less *immediate* danger; as the internal *Psora* that has sprung up in the whole organism has not yet had time to grow up to a high degree, and we must confess that the expulsion of a few vesicles of itch, that have just arisen, often shows no *immediate*, manifestly strong, evil consequences. Wherefore with delicate and aristocratic persons, or their children, it usually remains unknown, that a single vesicle or a few vesicles itching violently, which showed only a few days and were at once treated by the careful physician with Lead ointment or a Lotion of Lead, and which disappeared the following day, had itch for their foundation.

However small the internal *Psora* may be at the time of the quick suppression of an itch-eruption, which has only developed a few vesicles and which is then followed by only moderate ailments and complaints (which are then usually, from ignorance, ascribed by the domestic physician to other causes of little import): the internal malady of *Psora*, although as yet of slight degree, remains in its character and in its chronic nature the same general psoric disease of the whole organism; *i. e., without the aid of art it is ineradicable, and cannot be extirpated by the strength of even the best and most robust bodily constitution, and it will increase even to the end of the patient's life.* It is usually the case, indeed, that this disease, deprived as early as possible of the first traces of its cutaneous symptom by local applications, will grow but slowly in the beginning and will make but slow progress in the organism—much slower progress than where the eruption has been allowed to remain for a long time on the skin; for in the latter case the progress of the internal *Psora* is of immense rapidity; but the disease, nevertheless, increases unceasingly, and even in the best cases and uder the most favorable external circumstances, quietly and often for years unperceived by the eyes; so that anyone, who does not know the signs of its latent presence, would suppose and declare such persons to be healthy·and free from any internal malady. Often for years it does not manifest diseases.

Many hundred observations have gradually acquainted me* with the signs, by which the internally

* It was more easy to me, than to many hundreds of others, to find out and to recognize the signs of the *Psora* as well when latent and as yet slumbering within, as when it has grown to considerable chronic diseases, by an accurate comparison of the state of health of all such persons with myself, who, as is seldom the case, have never been afflicted with the *Psora* , and have, therefore, from my birth even until now in my eightieth year, been entirely free from the (smaller and greater) ailments enumerated here and further below, although I have been, on the whole, very apt to catch acute epidemic diseases, and have been exposed to many mental exertions and thousand fold vexations of spirit.

slumbering,* hitherto latent *Psora* (itch-malady) may be recognized even in those cases where it has not yet manifested itself in any startling disease, so that I am able to root out and to thoroughly cure this malady with its roots, more easily before the internal *Psora* has risen to a manifest (chronic) disease, and has developed to such a fearful height that the dangerous conditions make the cure difficult and in some cases impossible.

There are many signs of the *Psora* which is gradually increasing within, but is as yet slumbering, and has not yet come to the full outbreak of a manifest disease; but no one person has all these symptoms; the one has more of them, the other a smaller number; the one has at present only one of them, but in the course of time he will also have others; he may be free from some, according to the peculiar disposition of his body

---

*Allopathy has also assumed *hidden* (*latent*) conditions of disease in patients, in order to explain, or, at least, to excuse its blind inroads with violent medicines, blood-letting, anodynes, etc. These so-called *qualitates occultæ Fernelii* are, however, wholly suppositious and imaginary, as (according to the statement of this same physician) they are supposed not to be recognizable by any manifestations and symptoms. But whatever does not make known its hidden, imaginary existence by any sign does not exist for us men, who are limited by our Creator in our cognizance of things to observations—it is consequently a phantom of a roving fancy. It is quite different with the various forces *slumbering* (*latent*) in nature; despite their ordinary occultness, they, nevertheless, show themselves when the requisite circumstances and conditions appear; *e. g.*, latent heat, even in metals that feel cold, is manifested when they are rubbed, just as the *Psora* manifests itself; *e. g.*, as a drawing pain in the sheaths of the muscles, when the person infected with *Psora* has been exposed to a draught, etc.

or according to the external circumstances of different persons.

SYMPTOMS OF LATENT PSORA.

Mostly with children; frequent discharge of ascarides and other worms; unsufferable itching caused by the latter in the rectum.

The abdomen often distended.

Now insatiable hunger, then again want of appetite.

Paleness of the face and relaxation of the muscles.

Frequent inflammations of the eyes.

Swellings of the cervical glands (scrofula).

Perspiration on the head in the evening after going to sleep.

Epistaxis with girls and youths (more rarely with older persons), often very severe.

Usually cold hands or perspiration on the palms (burning in the palms).

Cold, dry or ill-smelling, sweaty feet (burning in the soles of the feet).

The arms or hands, the legs or feet, are benumbed by a slight cause.

Frequent cramps in the calves (the muscles of the arms and hands).

Painless subsultus of various portions of the muscles here and there on the body.

Frequent or tedious dry or fluent coryza or catarrh,* or impossibility of catching a cold even from the most

*The epidemic catarrhal fevers and catarrhs, which seize almost everyone, even the healthiest persons (Grippe, Influenza), do not belong to this category.

severe exposure, even while otherwise having continually ailments of this kind.

Long-continued obstruction of one or both nostrils.

Ulcerated nostrils (sore nose).

Disagreeable sensation of dryness in the nose.

Frequent inflammation of the throat, frequent hoarseness.

Short tussiculation in the morning.

Frequent attacks of dyspnœa.

Predisposition to catching cold (either in the whole body or only in the head, the throat, the breast, the abdomen, the feet; *e. g.*, in a draught,* (usually when these parts are inclined to perspiration), and many other, sometimes long-continuing ailments arising therefrom.

Predisposition to strains, even from carrying or lifting a slight weight, often caused even by stretching upward and reaching out the arms for objects which are hung high (so also a multitude of complaints resulting from a moderate stretching of the muscles, headache, nausea, prostration, tensive pain in the muscles of the neck and back, etc.).

Frequent one-sided headache or toothache, even from moderate emotional disturbances.

Frequent flushes of heat and redness of the face, not unfrequently with anxiety.

Frequent falling out of hair of the head, dryness of the same, many scales upon the scalp.

Predisposition to erysipelas now and then.

---

*Persons not afflicted with *Psora*, though draughts and damp cold air may not be agreeable to them, do not suffer any colds or evil after-effects therefrom.

Amenorrhœa, irregularities in the menses, too copious, too scanty, too early (too late), of too long duration, too watery, connected with various bodily ailments.

Twitching of the limbs on going to sleep.

Weariness early on awaking; unrefreshing sleep.

Perspiration in the morning in bed.

Perspiration breaks out too easily during the daytime, even with little movement (or inability to bring out perspiration).

White, or at least very pale tongue; still more frequently cracked tongue.

Much phlegm in the throat.

Bad smell from the mouth, frequently or almost constantly, especially early in the morning and during the menses, and this is perceived either as insipid, or as slightly sour, or as if from a stomach out of order, or as mouldy, also as putrid.

Sour taste in the mouth.

Nausea in the morning.

Sensation of emptiness in the stomach.

Repugnance to cooked, warm food especially to meat (principally with children).

Repugnance to milk.

At night or in the morning, dryness in the mouth.

Cutting pains in the abdomen, frequently or daily (especially with children), more frequently in the morning.

Hard stools, delaying usually more than a day, clotted, often covered with mucus (or nearly always soft, fermenting stools, like diarrhœa).

Venous knots on the anus; passage of blood with the stools.

Passing of mucus from the anus, with or without fæces.

Itching on the anus.

Dark urine.

Swollen, enlarged veins on the legs (swollen veins, varices).

Chilblains and pains as from chilblains, even outside of the severe cold of winter, even, also, in summer.

Pains as of corns, without any external pinching of the shoes.

Disposition to crack, strain or wrench one joint or another.

Cracking of one or more joints on moving.

Drawing, tensive pains in the neck, the back, the limbs, especially, also, in the teeth (in damp, stormy weather, in northwest and northeast winds, after colds, overlifting, disagreeable emotions, etc.).

Renewal of pains and complaints while at rest, and disappearance of the same while in motion.

Most of the ailments come on at night, and are increased with a low barometer, with north and northeast* winds, in winter and towards spring.

Uneasy, frightful, or at least too vivid, dreams.

Unhealthy skin; every little lesion passes into sores; cracked skin of the hands and of the lower lips.

Frequent boils, frequent felons (whitlows).

Dry skin on the limbs; on the arms, the thighs, and also at times on the cheeks.

Here or there a rough, scaling spot on the skin, which causes at times a voluptuous itching and, after the rubbing, a burning sensation.

In Europe northeast winds are cold, sharp and dry, corresponding to our west winds.—*Transl.

Here or there at times, though seldom, a single insufferably pleasant, but unbearably itching vesicle, at its point sometimes filled with pus, and causing a burning sensation after rubbing, on a finger, on the wrist or in some other place.

Suffering from several or from a greater number of these ailments (even at various times and frequently), a person will still consider himself as healthy, and is supposed to be so by others. He may also lead a quite endurable life in such a state and, without much hindrance, attend to his business as long as he is young or still in his vigorous years, and so long as he does not suffer any particular mishap from without, has a satisfactory income, does not live in vexation or grief, does not overexert himself; but especially if he is of quite a cheerful, equable, patient, contented disposition. With such persons the *Psora* (internal itch malady), which may be recognized by a connoisseur by means of a few or by more of the above symptoms, may slumber on for many years within, without causing any continuing chronic disease.

But still, even in such favorable external relations, as soon as these persons advance in age, even moderate causes (a slight vexation, or a cold, or an error in diet, etc.) may produce *a violent attack of (however only a brief) disease:* a violent attack of colic, inflammation of the chest or the throat, erysipelas, fever and the like, and the violence of these attacks seems to be out of proportion to its moderate cause. This is mostly wont to happen in fall or winter, but often also by preference in springtime.

But even where a person, whether a child or an

adult, who has the *Psora* slumbering within him, shows much semblance of health, but happens upon the opposite of the above-described favorable conditions of life, when his health and whole organism have been very much weakened and shaken by a prevalent epidemic fever or an infectious acute disease,* smallpox, measles, whooping cough, scarlet fever, purple rash, etc., or through an external severe lesion, a shock, a fall, a wound, a considerable burn, the breaking of an arm or a leg, a hard labor, the confinement due to a disease (*usually helped on by the incorrect and weakening allopathic treatment*), confinement at a sedentary occupation in a gloomy, close room, weakening the vital force; the sad losses of beloved relatives bending down the soul with grief, or daily vexation and annoyance, which embitter the life; deterioration of the food or an entire want of what is necessary and indispensable, exposure and inferior food beating down man's courage and strength; then the *Psora*, which has hitherto slumbered, awakes and shows itself in the heightened and augmented symptoms enumerated below, in its transition to the formation of severe maladies; one or another nameless (psoric) chronic dis-

---

*At the termination of an acute fever there often follows, as if incited by such a fever, an appearance of an old *Psora* residing in the body, as an eruption of itch. This the physicians explain as a new generation of itch in this individual body replete with bad humors (*scilicet*), since they know nothing of a *Psora* in man which may be quiescent for a long period. But the itch-disease cannot now be generated or arise or be created anew of itself, just as no smallpox or cowpox, no measles, no venereal chancre disease, etc., can now make its appearance with any man without previous infection.

eases* breaks out and, *most of all, through weakening and exhausting improper treatment by allopathic physicians*, they are aggravated from time to time without intermission, often to a fearful height, if external circumstances favorable for the patient do not interpose, and cause a moderation in the process of the malady.

---

*The one or the other disease, according to the original bodily constitution, a peculiar mode of living, a peculiar disposition of the mind, often arising from the individual education or a more receptive or more weakened condition of some part of the body, gives a peculiar direction to the disease, and thus causes the itch disease to lead to the origin of the one or the other disease, so as to show itself preferably in that one direction and develop itself in that particular modification. A passionate, peevish disposition gives an extraordinary predisposition to the development of the *Psora;* so, also, previous exhaustion through frequent pregnancies, excessive nursing of infants, extraordinary hardships, *exhausting erroneous medical treatment*, debauchery, and a profligate mode of living. The internal itch disease is, as before mentioned, of such a peculiar nature that it may remain, as it were, tied down and covered up for a long time through external favorable surroundings, so that a man may seem to the superficial observer healthy for years, even for many years, until circumstances unfavorable to the body or the soul, or to both, may arise and serve as a hostile impulse to awaken the disease slumbering within and thus develop its germs. His acquaintances and his physician, yea, the patient himself, can not thon comprehend how his health could so suddenly fall into a decline. To bring some examples for explanation from my own experience: After a simple fracture of a limb attended with confinement to bed for five or six weeks, there may follow diseased conditions of another kind, the cause of which cannot be guessed, which diseased conditions, even when measurably removed, nevertheless return, and which, even without any error in diet, nevertheless at their return show aggravation. This is mostly the case in fall (winter) and spring and becomes a tedious ailment increasing from year to year, a lasting cure for which, without the substitution of a

But even if favorable external conditions should gain check the rapid development of a disease that

---

still worse disease for it by an allopathic cure, has been hitherto vainly sought for in the councils of former physicians and also in visits to mineral springs. There are in man's life innumerable stumbling-blocks or unfavorable occurrences of this kind which serve to awaken the *Psora* (the internal itch-disease), which till then has been slumbering (perhaps for a long time previously), and which cause its germs to develop. They are often of such a nature that the grave evils which gradually follow on them are out of all proportion to them, so that no rational man can consider those occurrences as sufficient causes for the chronic diseases which follow and which are often of a fearful character. But such a man is compelled to acknowledge a deeper seated hostile cause of these appearances, which cause has only now developed itself.

For example, a young married woman, who, viewed superficially and according to the common standard, was healthy, but who had in her childhood been infected with *Psora*, had the misfortune to be thrown out of her carriage while in the third month of her pregnancy, from which she suffered not only slight injury and the fright, but also a miscarriage, and the attending loss of blood gave her a considerable set-back. In a few weeks, however, her youthful constitution had pretty well recovered, and she might have been assured of a speedy return to lasting good health, when the announcement of the dangerous illness of a beloved sister, living at a distance, threw her back and augmented her former ailments, which had not yet been quite removed, by the addition of a multitude of nervous disorders and convulsions, thus turning them into a serious illness. Better news from her sister, indeed, followed, and at last good news. At last her sister, entirely restored herself, pays her a visit. But the sick young wife still remains sick, and even if she seems to recover for a week or two, her ailments nevertheless return without any apparent cause. Every succeeding confinement, even when quite easy, every hard winter, adds new ailments to the old, or the former disorders change into others still more troublesome, so that at last there ensues a serious chronic illness, though no one can see why the full vigor of youth, attended by

has broken out, true health can not be lastingly restored by any of the modes of treatment hitherto

---

happy external surroundings, should not have soon wiped out the consequence of that one miscarriage; still less can it be explained why the unfortunate impression of those sad tidings should not have disappeared on hearing of the recovery of her sister, or at least on the actual presence of her sister fully restored.

If the cause must at all times be proportionate to its effect and consequence, as is the case in nature, no one can see how, after the removal of the causes assailing her health, the resulting ailments could not only continue, but even increase from year to year, if their cause were not in something else, something deeper, so that those unhappy occurrences (the miscarriage and the sad tidings), since they both disappeared of themselves and therefore could not possibly yield a sufficient ground for the ensuing chronic disease, can only be regarded as the occasion, but not the efficient cause, of the development of a hostile power of greater importance pre-existent in the internal organism, but hitherto quiescent.

In a similar manner, a robust merchant, apparently healthy, despite some traces of internal *Psora*, perceptible only to the professional examiner, may, in consequence of unlucky commercial conjunctures, become involved in his finances, even so as to approach bankruptcy, and at the same time he will fall gradually into various ailments and finally into serious illness. The death of a rich kinsman, however, and the gaining of a great prize in a lottery, abundantly cover his commercial losses; he becomes a man of means—but his illness, nevertheless, not only continues, but increases from year to year, despite all medical prescriptions, in spite of his visiting the most famous baths, or rather, perhaps, with the assistance of these two causes.

A modest girl, who, excepting some signs of internal *Psora*, was accounted quite healthy, was compelled into a marriage which made her unhappy of soul, and in the same degree her bodily health declined, without any trace of venereal infection. No allopathic medicine alleviates her sad ailments, which continually grow more threatening. But in the midst of this aggravation, after one year's suffering, the cause of her unhappiness, her hated hus-

known, and the customary allopathic treatments, with their aggressive, inappropriate remedies—such as baths, Mercury, Prussic acid, Iodine, Digitalis, Qui-

---

band, is taken from her by death, and she seems to revive, in the conviction that she is now delivered from every occasion of mental or bodily illness, and hopes for a speedy recovery; all her friends hope the same for her, as the exciting cause of her illness lies in the grave. She also improves speedily, but unexpectedly she still remains an invalid, despite the vigor of her youth; yea, her ailments but seldom leave her, and are renewed from time to time without any external cause, and they are even aggravated from year to year in the rough months.

A person who had been unjustly suspected and become involved in a serious criminal suit, and who had before seemed healthy, with the exception of the marks of latent *Psora* mentioned above, during these harassing months fell into various diseased states. But finally the innocence of the accused is acknowledged, and an honorable acquittal followed. We might suppose that such a happy, gratifying event would necessarily give new life to the accused and remove all bodily complaints. But this does not take place, the person still at times suffers from these ailments, and they are even renewed with longer or briefer intermissions, and are aggravated with the passing years, especially in the wintry seasons.

How shall we explain this? If that disagreeable event had been the cause, the *sufficient* cause, of these ailments, ought not the effect, *i. e.*, the disease, to have entirely ceased of necessity after the removal of the cause? But these ailments do not cease, they are in time renewed and even gradually aggravated, and it becomes evident that those disagreeable events could not have been the sufficient cause of the present ailments and complaints—it is seen that they *only served as an occasion and impetus toward the development of a malady, which till then only slumbered within.*

The recognition of this old internal foe, which is so frequently present, and the science which is able to overcome it, make it manifest that generally an indwelling itch disease (*Psora*) was the ground of all these ailments, which can not be overcome even by the vigor of the best constitution, but only through art.

nine, starvation and other fashionable remedies included—only hasten death, the end of all those maladies which the physician cannot heal.

When once, under the above-mentioned unfavorable outward surroundings, the transition of the *Psora* from its slumbering and bound condition to its awakening and outbreak has taken place, and the patient leaves himself to the injurious activity of the usual allopathic physician, who deems it appropriate to his office and his income to mercilessly assault the organism of the patient (as we are sorry to witness every day) with the battering-rams of his violent, inappropriate remedies and weakening treatments;—in such a case, the external circumstances of the patient and his situation with respect to his surroundings may have changed ever so favorably, but the aggravation of the disease nevertheless proceeds under such hands without any escape.

The awakening of the internal *Psora* which has hitherto slumbered and been latent, and, as it were, kept bound by a good bodily constitution and favorable external circumstances, as well as its breaking out into more serious ailments and maladies, is announced by the increase of the symptoms given above as indicating the slumbering *Psora*, and also by a numberless multitude of various other signs and complaints. These are varied according to the difference in the bodily constitution of a man, his hereditary disposition, the various errors in his education and habits, his manner of living and diet, his employments, his turn of mind, his morality, etc.

Then when the itch-malady develops into a manifest secondary disease there appear the following symptoms, which I have derived and observed altogether from accounts of diseases which I myself have treated successfully and which confessedly originated from the contagion of itch, and were mixed neither with syphilis nor sycosis.

I am quite willing to believe that many more symptoms may have occurred in the experience of others.

I would only add further, that among the symptoms adduced there are also such as are entirely opposed to each other, the reason of which may be found in the varying bodily constitutions existing at the time—when the outbreak of the internal *Psora* occurred. Yet the one variety of symptoms is found more rarely than the other and it offers no particular obstruction to a cure:

Vertigo ; reeling while walking.

Vertigo ; when closing the eyes, everything seems to turn around with him ; he is at the same time seized with nausea.

Vertigo ; on turning around briskly, he almost falls over.

Vertigo, as if there was a jerk in the head, which causes a momentary loss of consciousness.

Vertigo with frequent eructations.

Vertigo even when only looking down on the level ground, or when looking upward.

Vertigo while walking on a road not enclosed on either side, in an open plain.

Vertigo ; she seems to herself now too large, now too small, or other objects have this appearance to her.

Vertigo, resembling a swoon.

Vertigo, passing over into unconsciousness.

Dizziness; inability to think or to perform mental labor.

Her thoughts are not under her control.

She is at times quite without thought (sits lost in thought).

The open air causes dizziness and drowsiness in the head.

Everything at times seems dark and black before his eyes, while walking or stooping, or when raising himself from a stooping posture.

Rush of blood to the head.[1]

Heat in the head (and in the face).[2]

A cold pressure on the top of the head.[3]

Headache, a dull pain in the morning immediately on waking up, or in the afternoon when walking rapidly or speaking loudly.

Headache on one side, with a certain periodicity (after 28, 14 or a less number of days), more frequently during full moon, or during the new moon, or after mental excitement, after a cold, etc.; a pressure or other pain on top of the head or inside of it, or a boring pain over one of the eyes.[4]

---

[1] While the mind is uneasy, with anxiety and disinclination to work.

[2] Not unfrequently accompanied with coldness of the hands and feet.

[3] Usually accompanied with anxiety.

[4] At the same time a great internal disquiet and anxiety, especially in the abdomen; a lack of stools, or frequent, scanty evacuations attended with anxiety; heaviness in the limbs, quivering in the whole body, tension of all the nerves with great irritability and sensitiveness; the eye can not bear any light, lachrymation,

Headache daily at certain hours; *e. g.*, a stitching in the temples.[1]

Attacks of throbbing headache (*e. g.*, in the forehead) with violent nausea as if about to sink down, or, also, vomiting; starting early in the evenings, repeated every fortnight, or sooner or later.

Headache as if the skull were about to burst open.[2]

Headache, drawing pains.[3]

Headache, stitches in the head (passing out at the ears).[4]

Roaring noise in the brain, singing, buzzing, humming, thundering, etc.

The scalp full of dandruff, with or without itching.

Eruption on the head, tinea capitis, malignant tinea with crusts of greater or less thickness, with sensitive

---

sometimes with swelling of the eyes; the feet are cold; at times attended with dry coryza; often chills, then again a flying heat; conjoined with this, continuous nausea, also at times, retching and vomiting; she lies either as if stunned, or throws herself anxiously from side to side, the attacks lasting from twelve to twenty-four and more hours. After these attacks either great weariness with sadness, or a feeling of tension all over the body. Before these attacks there are frequent jerks of the limbs during sleep and starting up from sleep, anxious dreams, gnashing of the teeth in sleep and tendency to start at any sudden noise.

[1] Which also swell at times, with lachrymation of the one eye.

[2] In some cases a drawing pain from the nape of the neck toward the occiput, at times also all over the whole head and face, which is often bloated from it, while the head aches when touched, not infrequently attended with nausea.

[3] Usually while walking, especially while walking and moving after meals.

[4] At the same time everything frequently appears dark before her face.

stitches when one of the places becomes moist; when it becomes moist a violent itching; the whole crown of the head painfully sensitive to the open air; with it hard swellings of the glands in the neck.

The hair of the head as if parched.

The hair of the head frequently falls out, most in front, on the crown and top of the head; bald spots or beginning baldness of certain spots.

Under the skin are formed painful lumps, which come and pass away, like bumps and round tumors.[1]

Feeling of contraction in the skin of the scalp and the face.

Paleness of the face during the first sleep, with blue rings around the eyes.

Frequent redness of the face, and heat.[2]

Yellowish; yellow color of the face.

Sallow yellowish complexion.

Erysipelas on the face.[3]

Pressive pain on the eyes, especially late in the evening; he must shut them.

He cannot look long at anything, else everything flickers before him; objects seem to move.

The eyelids, especially in the morning, are as if closed; he cannot open them (for minutes; yea, even

---

[1] Which also in rare cases pass over into suppuration.

[2] He at times also becomes quite weak and weary from it or anxious, and he perspires on the upper part of the body; his eyes at times become dim; everything becomes black before his eyes, his mind is sad; his head also feels as if too full with burning in the temples.

[3] In some cases with much fever, also at times with burning, itching, stinging watery blisters in the face, which turn into scabs (Erysipelas bullosum).

for hours); the eye-lids are heavy as if paralyzed or convulsively closed.

The eyes are most sensitive to daylight; they are pained by it and close involuntarily.[1]

Sensation of cold in the eyes.

The canthi are full of pus-like mucus (eye-gum).

The edges of the eyelids full of dry mucus.

On the edges of the eyelids, inflammation of single Meibomian glands or several of them.

Inflammations of the eyes, of various kinds.[2]

Yellowness around the eyes.

Yellowness of the white of the eye.

Dim, opaque spots on the cornea.[4]

Dropsy of the eye.

Obscuration of the crystalline lens, cataract.

Squinting.

Far-sightedness; he sees far in the distance, but cannot clearly distinguish small objects held close.

Short-sightedness; he can see even small objects by holding them close to the eye, but the more distant the object is the more indistinct it appears, and at a great distance he does not see it.

False vision; he sees objects double, or manifold, or only the one-half of them.

Before his eyes there are floating as it were flies, or black points, or dark streaks, or networks, especially when looking into bright daylight.

---

[1] Usually with more or less inflammation.

[2] The *fistula lachrymalis* has probably never any other cause than the itching disease.

[3] Or gray color of the same.

[4] Even without having had any previous inflammation of the eyes.

The eyes seem to look through a veil or a mist; the sight becomes dim at certain times.

Night-blindness; he sees well in daytime, but in the twilight he cannot see at all.

Blindness by day; he can only see well during the twilight.

Amaurosis; uninterrupted dimness of vision[1] increased finally even to blindness.

Painfulness of various spots in the face, the cheeks, the cheekbones, the lower jaw, etc., when touched; while chewing, as if festering inwardly; also like stitches and jerks; especially in chewing there are jerks, stitches and a tension so that he cannot eat.[2]

The hearing is excessively irritated and sensitive; she cannot bear to hear a bell ring without trembling; he is thrown into convulsions by the beating of the drum, etc.; many sounds cause pains in the ear.

There are stitches in the ear, outwardly.[3]

Crawling sensation and itching in the ear.

Dryness in the ear; dry scabs within, without any ear-wax.

Running from the ear of thin, usually ill-smelling pus.

Pulsation in the ear.

Various sounds and noises in the ear.[4]

---

[1] More frequently without opacity of the crystalline lens than with it.

[2] During chewing or speaking there is at times also a similar twitching on the sides of the head, where protuberances like painful bumps often arise. When the pain is still more unbearable and at times combined with a burning pain, it is called Fothergill's pain in the face.

[3] Especially while walking in the open air.

[4] Such as clinking, rushing, seething, roaring, humming, chirp-

Deafness of various degrees even up to total deafness, with or without noise in the ear; occasionally worse, according to the weather.

Swelling of the parotid glands.[1]

Epistaxis, more or less profusely, more or less frequently.

The nostrils as it were stopped up.[2]

Sensation of dryness in the nose, troublesome even when the air passes freely.

Polypi of the nose (usually with the loss of the power of smelling); these may extend also through the nasal passages into the fauces.

Sense of smell, weak, lost.

Sense of smell perverted.[3]

Too violent sensation of smell, higher and highest sensitiveness for even imperceptible odors.

Scabs in the nose; discharge of pus or hardened clots of mucus.[4]

Fetid smell in the nose.

Nostrils frequently ulcerated, surrounded with pimples and scabs.

Swelling and redness of the nose or the tip of the nose, frequent or continual.

Under the nose, or on the upper lip, long-lasting scabs or itching pimples.

---

ing, ringing, drumming, thundering, whizzing, fluttering, murmuring, etc.

[1] Often with stinging pains in the glands.

[2] Either one or both, or alternately, first one, then the other; often there is only the sensation of being stopped up, while the air can be freely drawn in through it.

[3] *E.g.*, the smell of manure or some other peculiar smell is in the nose.

[4] Sometimes also a discharge of acrid mucus from the nose.

The red of the lips is quite pale.

The red of the lips is dry, scabby, peeling off; it chaps.

Swelling of the lips, especially of the upper lip.[1]

The inside of the lips is lined with little sores or blisters.[2]

Cutaneous eruption of the beard and of the roots of the hairs of the beard, with itching.

Eruptions of the face of innumerable kinds.[3]

Glands of the lower jaw swollen, sometimes passing over into chronic suppuration.

Glandular swellings down the sides of the neck.

Gums bleeding at a slight touch.

Gums, the external or the internal, painful, as if from wounds.

Gums, with erosive itching.

Gums, whitish, swollen, painful on touching.

Gums, recession, leaving the front teeth and their roots bare.

Gnashing of the teeth during sleep.

Looseness of the teeth, and many kinds of deterioration of the teeth, even without toothache.

Toothache of innumerable varieties, with varying causes of excitation.

She cannot remain in bed at night, owing to toothache.

On the tongue, painful blisters and sore places.

---

[1] At times with a burning, biting pain.

[2] Often very painful, coming and passing away.

[3] Milk-crust, pimples, blotches, herpes and carcinomatous ulcers of the nose, lips and face (also called *cancer*), with burning and stinging pain.

Tongue white, coated white or furred white.

Tongue pale, bluish-white.

Tongue full of deep furrows ; here and there, as if torn above.

Tongue dry.

Sensation of dryness on the tongue, even while it is properly moist.

Stuttering, stammering; also at times sudden attacks of inability to speak.

On the inside of the cheeks painful blisters or sores.

Flow of blood from the mouth; often severe.

Sensation of dryness of the whole internal mouth, or merely in spots, or deep down in the throat.[1]

Fetid smell from the mouth.

Burning in the throat.

Constant flow of saliva, especially while speaking, particularly in the morning.

Continual spitting of saliva.

Frequent mucus deep down in the throat (the fauces), which he has to hawk up and expectorate frequently during the day, especially in the morning.

Frequently inflammation of the throat, and swelling of the parts used in swallowing.

Insipid, slimy taste in the mouth.

Intolerably sweet taste in the mouth, almost constantly.

Bitter taste in the mouth, mostly in the morning.[2]

---

[1] Chiefly on waking up at night or in the morning, with or without thirst; with a great deal of dryness in the throat, often a pricking pain in swallowing.

[2] Not rarely, this is constant.

Sourish and sour taste in the mouth, especially after eating, though the food tasted all right.[1]

Putrid and fetid taste in the mouth.

Bad smell in the mouth, sometimes mouldy, sometimes putrid like old cheese, or like fetid foot-sweat, or like rotten sour kraut.

Eructations, with the taste of the food, several hours after eating.

Eructations, empty, loud, of mere air, uncontrollable, often for hours, not infrequently at night.

Incomplete eructation, which causes merely convulsive shocks in the fauces without coming out of the mouth.

Eructation, sour, either fasting or after food, especially after milk.

Eructation, which excites to vomiting.

Eructation, rancid (especially after eating fat things).

Eructation, putrid or mouldy, early in the morning.

Frequent eructations before meals, with a sort of rabid hunger.

Heart-burn, more or less frequent; there is a burning along the chest, especially after breakfast, or while moving the body.

Water-brash, a gushing discharge of a sort of salivary fluid from the stomach, preceded by writhing pains in the stomach (the pancreas), with a sensation of weakness (shakiness), nausea causing as it were a swoon, and gathering of the saliva in the mouth, even at night.[2]

---

[1] Rarely an offensively sweet taste in the mouth, even without eating or drinking.

[2] This also at times turns into vomiting of water, mucus, or a

The ruling complaints in any part of the body are excited after eating fresh fruit, especially if this is acidulous, also after Acetic acid (in salads, etc.).

Nausea early in the morning.[1]

Nausea even to vomiting, in the morning immediately after rising from bed, decreasing from motion.

Nausea always after eating fatty things or milk.

Vomiting blood.

Hiccough after eating or drinking.

Swallowing impeded by spasms, even causing a man to die of hunger.

Spasmodic, involuntary swallowing.

Frequent sensation of fasting and of emptiness in the stomach (or abdomen), not unfrequently with much saliva in the mouth.

Ravenous hunger (canine hunger), especially early in the morning; he has to eat at once else he grows faint, exhausted and shaky (or if he is in the open air he has to lie straight down).

Ravenous hunger with rumbling and grumbling in the abdomen.

Appetite without hunger; she has a desire to swallow down in haste various things without there being any craving therefor in the stomach.

A sort of hunger; but when she then eats ever so little, she feels at once satiated and full.

When she wants to eat, she feels full in the chest and her throat feels as if full of mucus.

---

gush of acrid acid—more frequently after eating flour dumplings, vegetables causing flatulence, baked prunes, etc.

[1] Often coming very suddenly.

Want of appetite; only a sort of gnawing, turning and writhing in the stomach urges her to eat.

Repugnance to cooked, warm food, especially to boiled meat, and hardly any longing for anything but rye-bread (with butter), or for potatoes.[1]

In the morning, at once, thirst; constant thirst.

In the pit of the stomach there is a sensation of swelling, painful to the touch.

Sensation of coldness in the pit of the stomach.

Pressure in the stomach or in the pit of the stomach, as from a stone, or a constricting pain (cramp).[2]

In the stomach, beating and pulsation, even when fasting.

Spasm in the stomach; pain in the pit of the stomach as if drawn together.[3]

Griping in the stomach; a painful griping in the stomach;[4] it suddenly constricts the stomach, especially after cold drinking.

Pain in the stomach, as if sore, when eating even the most harmless kinds of foods.

Pressure in the stomach, even when fasting, but more from every kind of food, or from particular dishes, fruit, green vegetables, rye-bread, food containing vinegar, etc.[5]

---

[1] Especially in youth and childhood.

[2] In some cases even while fasting, and causing him to wake up out of sleep at night, sometimes oppressing the breathing.

[3] Usually a short time after eating.

[4] Not infrequently with vomiting of mucus and water, without which in such a case the griping is not alleviated.

[5] Even after partaking of the slightest quantity of such things, there may also ensue colic, pain or numbness of the jaws, tearing pain in the teeth, copious accumulation of mucus in the throat, etc.

During eating, feels dizzy and giddy, threatening to fall to one side.

After the slightest supper, nocturnal heat in bed; in the morning, constipation and exceeding lassitude.

After meals, anxiety and cold perspiration, with anxiety.[1]

During eating, perspiration.

Immediately after eating, vomiting.

After meals, pressure and burning in the stomach, or in the epigastrium, almost like heartburn.

After eating, burning in œsophagus from below upward.

After meals, distension of the abdomen.[2]

After meals, very tired and sleepy.[3]

After meals, as if intoxicated.

After meals, headache.

After meals, palpitation of the heart.

Alleviation of several, even remote, complaints from eating.

The flatus does not pass off, but moves about, causing many ailments of body and of spirit.[4]

---

[1] There may also be pains, renewed now and then; *e. g.*, stitches in the lips, griping and digging in the abdomen, pressure in the chest, heaviness in the back and the small of the back, even to nausea; when nothing but an artificially excited vomiting will give relief. With some the anguish is aggravated after eating, even to an impulse to destroy themselves by strangulation.

[2] With this, at times, weariness in the arms and legs.

[3] Often until the patient lies down and sleeps.

[4] At times drawing pains in the limbs, especially in the lower limbs, or stitches in the pit of the stomach, or in the side of the abdomen, etc.

The abdomen is distended by flatus,[1] the abdomen feels full, especially after a meal.

Sensation as if the flatus ascended; followed by eructations—then often a sensation of burning in the throat, or vomiting by day and by night.

Pain in the hypochondria when touched, and in motion, or also during rest.

Constricting pain in the epigastrium, immediately under the ribs.

Cutting pains in the abdomen, as if from obstructed flatus; there is a constant sensation of fulness in the abdomen—the flatus rises upwards.

Cutting pains in the abdomen almost daily, especially with children, oftener in the morning than in other parts of the day, sometimes day and night, without diarrhœa.

Cutting pains in the abdomen, especially on the one side of the abdomen, or the groin.[2]

In the abdomen, qualmishness, a sensation of voidness, disagreeable emptiness;[3] even immediately after eating, he felt as if he had not eaten anything.

From the small of the back, around the abdomen, especially below the stomach, a sensation of constriction as from a bandage, after she had had no stool for several days.

---

[1] The flatus often ascends; less frequently a great quantity of flatus is discharged, especially in the morning, without smell and without alleviating the other ailments; in other cases flatulence, with a great quantity of excessively fetid flatus passing off.

[2] The cutting pain also at times passes down into the rectum and down the thigh.

[3] In some cases alternating with a contractive pain in the abdomen.

Pain in the liver, when touching the right side of the abdomen.

Pain in the liver, a pressure and tension—a tension below the ribs on the right side.

Below the last ribs (in the hypochondria), a tension and pressure all over, which checks the breathing and makes the mind anxious and sad.

Pain in the liver, stitches—mostly when stooping quickly.

Inflammation of the liver.

Pressure in the abdomen as from a stone.[1]

Hardness of the abdomen.

Crampy colic, a grasping pain in the bowels.

In colic, coldness on one side of the abdomen.

A clucking, croaking and audible rumbling and grumbling in the abdomen.[2]

So-called uterine spasms, like labor pains, grasping pains often compelling the patient to lie down, frequently quickly distending the abdomen without flatulence.

In the lower abdomen, pains pressing down toward the genitals.[3]

Inguinal hernias, often painful while speaking and singing.[4]

---

[1] Which often rises to the pit of the stomach, digging and causing vomiting.

[2] At times only in the left side of the abdomen, passing upwards with the inspiration and downward with the expiration.

[3] Pressing down as if to cause a prolapsus, and when it is passed she feels heavy in all her limbs, the limbs go to sleep; she must stretch and extend her limbs.

[4] Inguinal hernias rise as a rule only from internal Psora, excepting the few cases, when these parts are injured by great ex-

Swellings of the inguinal glands, which sometimes turn into suppuration.

Constipation ; delayed stools sometimes for several days, not infrequently with repeated ineffectual urging to stool.

Stools hard, as if burnt, in small knots, like sheep-dung, often covered with mucus, sometimes also enveloped by veinlets of blood.

Stools of mere mucus (mucous piles).

Passage of round worms from the anus.

Discharge of pieces of tape-worm.

Stools, in the beginning very hard and troublesome, followed by diarrhœa.

Very pale, whitish stool.

Gray stools.

Green stools.

Clay-colored stools.

Stools with putrid, sour smell.

At the stools, cutting pains in the rectum.

Stools show diarrhœa for several weeks, months, years.[1]

Frequently repeated diarrhœa, with cutting pains in the abdomen, lasting several days.

After a stool, especially after a softer, more copious evacuation, great and sudden prostration.[2]

---

ternal violence, or when the hernia arises from superhuman exertions of the body through lifting or pushing quickly, while in a great fright.

[1] Usually preceded by rumbling or fermentation in the abdomen; chiefly in the morning.

[2] Especially, weakness in the pit of the stomach, anxiety, restlessness, also at times chills in the abdomen or the small of the back, etc.

Diarrhœa, soon so weakening, that she cannot walk alone.

Painless and painful hemorrhoidal varices[1] on the anus, in the rectum (blind piles).

Bleeding hemorrhoidal varices on the anus or in the rectum[2] (running piles), especially during stools, after which the hemorrhoids often pain violently for a long time.

With bloody discharges in the anus or in the rectum, ebullition of blood through the body and short breathing.

Formication and itching formication in the rectum, with or without the discharge of ascarides.

Itching and erosion in the anus and the perinæum.

Polypi in the rectum.

During micturition, anxiety, also at times prostration.

At times too much urine is discharged, succeeded by great weariness.[3]

Painful retention of urine (with children and old people).

When he is chilled (feels cold through and through), he cannot urinate.

At times owing to flatulence, she cannot urinate.

The urethra is constricted in parts, especially in the morning.

---

[1] Which not infrequently have a slimy fluid oozing from them.

[2] *Fistulæ in ano* have probably never any other cause than this malady, especially when to this there are added a stimulating diet, an excess in spirituous liquors, frequent laxatives, a sedentary occupation and abuse of the sexual instinct.

[3] *Diabetes*, which with Allopathic remedies is usually so fatal, has probably never any other origin than this malady.

[4] The urine frequently passes off as thin as a thread, or the

Pressure on the bladder, as if from an urging to urinate, immediately after drinking.

He cannot hold the urine for any length of time, it presses on the bladder, and passes off while he walks, sneezes, coughs or laughs.

Frequent micturition at night; he has to get up frequently at night for that purpose.

Urine passes off in sleep involuntarily.

After urinating, the urine continues to drip out for a long time.

Whitish urine, with a sweetish smell and taste, passes off in excessive abundance, with prostration, emaciation and inextinguishable thirst (diabetes).

During urination, burning, also lancinating pains in the urethra and the neck of the bladder.

Urine of penetrating, sharp odor.

The urine quickly deposits a sediment.

The urine discharged is at once turbid like whey.

With the urine there is discharged from time to time a red sand (kidney grits).

Dark-yellow urine.

Brown urine.

Blackish urine.

Urine with blood particles, also at times complete hematuria.

---

stream spreads out; the urine is only discharged in jerks at long intervals; these interruptions are frequently caused by a spasm in the neck of the bladder which antagonizes the action of the bladder and springs from the same Psoric malady. So also inflammation of the bladder from strictures of the urethra, and the *fistula in vesica* are always of Psoric origin, though in rare cases *sycosis* may be complicated with the *Psora*.

Discharge of prostatic fluid after urination, but especially after a difficult stool (also almost constant dripping of the same).[1]

Nocturnal passage of semen, too frequent, one, two or three times a week, or even every night.[2]

Nightly discharge of the genital fluid in a woman, with voluptuous dreams.

Nocturnal pollutions, even if not frequent, yet immediately attended by evil consequences.[3]

Semen passes off almost involuntarily in daytime, with little excitation, often even without erection.

Erections very frequent, long continuing, very painful without pollutions.

The semen is not discharged, even during a long-continued coition and with a proper erection,[4] but it passes off afterward in nocturnal pollutions or with the urine.

Accumulation of water in the tunica vaginalis of the testicle (hydrocele).

There is never a complete erection, even with the most voluptuous excitement.

---

[1] Sometimes also consumption from the constant oozing out of the prostatic fluid.

[2] With healthy chaste young men, pollutions naturally only take place every twelve or fourteen days, without any attending troubles, and they are followed by cheerfulness and a feeling of strength and serenity.

[3] Gloominess, obtuseness, dimness of the thinking powers, diminished vividness of the imagination, want of memory, depression, melancholy; the vision is weakened, as well as the digestion and the appetite; stools are retained, a rush of blood to the head ensues, also toward the anus etc.

[4] The testicles in such a case are never drawn up to the body, but hang down more or less.

Painful twitches in the muscles of the penis.

Itching of the scrotum, which is sometimes beset with pimples and scabs.

One or both of the testicles chronically swollen, or showing a knotty induration (*Sarcocele*).

Dwindling, diminution, disappearance of one or both testicles.

Induration and enlargement of the prostatic gland.

Drawing pain in the testicle and the spermatic chord.

Pain as from contusion in the testicle.

Lack of sexual desire in both sexes, either frequent or constant.[1]

Uncontrollable insatiable lasciviousness,[2] with a cachectic complexion and sickly body.

Sterility, impotence, without any original organic defect in the sexual parts.[3]

---

[1] Often for years, yea, for many years. The male and the female genital parts cannot then be excited to any agreeable or voluptuous sensation—the body of the male penis hangs down relaxed, is thinner than the glans penis, which feels cold and is of a bluish or white color; in the female parts the labia are not excitable, they are relaxed and small; the vagina almost numb and insensible, and usually dry; sometimes there is a falling out of the hair of the pudenda, or an entire bareness of the female genital parts.

[2] Metromania and Nymphomania are of the same origin.

[3] Too frequent coition from impotent lasciviousness, with too sudden a passing off of immature, watery semen, or lack of erection, or lack of the issue of semen, or lack of sexual desire—menses too copious, or a constant flow of blood; watery, scanty or deficient menses; copious discharge of mucus from the vagina (leucorrhœa), indurated ovaries, the breasts have either dwindled down or become knotty; insensibility, or merely painful sensibility of the genital organs, are merely the proximate usual symptoms of sterility or impotence with the one sex or the other.

Disorders of the menstrual function; the menses do not appear regularly on the twenty-eighth day after their last appearance, they do not come on without other ailments and not at once, and do not continue steadily for three or four days with a moderate quantity of healthy-colored, mild blood, until on the fourth day it imperceptibly comes to an end without any disturbance of the general health of body and spirit; nor are the menses continued to the forty-eighth or fiftieth year, nor do they cease gradually and without any troubles.

The menses are slow in setting in after the fifteenth year and later, or after appearing one or more times, they cease for several months and for years.[1]

The menses do not keep their regular periods, they either come several days too early, sometimes every three weeks, or even every fortnight.[2]

The menses flow only one day, only a few hours, or in imperceptibly small quantities.

The menses flow for five, six, eight and more days, but only intermittently, a little flow every six, twelve, twenty-four hours, and then they cease for half or whole days, before more is discharged.

The menses flow too strongly, for weeks, or return almost daily (bloody flux).[3]

---

[1] Consequent sallow paleness and tumefaction of the face, heaviness of the limbs, swelling of the feet, chilliness, weariness, asthma (chlorosis), etc.

[2] The menses rarely come several days too late, and flow then in too great abundance, with prostrating weariness and many other ailments.

[3] Often followed by swelling of the face, of the hands and feet,

Menses of watery blood or of brown clots of blood.

Menses of very fetid blood.

Menses accompanied with many ailments, swoons or (mostly stitching) headaches, or contractive, spasmodic, cutting pains in the abdomen and in the small of the back; she is obliged to lie down, vomit, etc.

Polypi in the vagina.

Leucorrhœa from the vagina, one or several days before, or soon after, the monthly flow of blood, or during the whole time from the one menstrual discharge to the other, with a diminution of the menses, or continuing solely instead of the menses; the flow is like milk, or like white, or yellow mucus, or like acrid, or sometimes like fetid, water.[1]

---

painful spasms in the breast and the abdomen, innumerable ailments from nervous debility, excessive sensitiveness, as well in general, as of particular sensory organs, etc., and before the appearance of the flow, anxious dreams, frequent awakenings with a rush of blood to the head, palpitation, restlessness, etc. With a more violent flow of blood from the uterus, there are often cutting pains in the one side of the abdomen and in the groin; the cutting pain sometimes descends into the rectum and into the thigh; then she frequently cannot urinate, or sit down, on account of her pains; after these pains the abdomen aches as if it were festering.

[1] Leucorrhœa, especially the more malignant kind, is accompanied by an innumerable multitude of ailments. Not to mention the lesser ones (such as the itching of the pudenda and the vagina, with excoriation on the outside of the pudenda and the adjacent part of the thigh, especially in walking), hysterical states of all kinds follow the more severe cases of this troublesome flux, as also disturbances of the mind and spirit, melancholy, insanity, epilepsy, etc. Often it comes in the form of an attack, and then it is preceded by a digging in the one side of the abdomen, or by burning in the stomach, in the lower abdomen, in the vagina or stitches in the vagina and in the mouth of the uterus, or a constrictive

Premature births.

During pregnancies great weariness, nausea, frequent vomiting, swoons, painful varicose veins on the thighs and the legs, and also at times on the labia, hysteric ailments of various kinds, etc.

Coryza at once, whenever she comes into the open air; then usually a stuffed coryza while in her room.

Dry coryza and a stuffed nose often, or almost constantly, also sometimes with intermissions.

Fluent coryza at the least taking of cold, therefore, mostly in the inclement season and when it is wet.

Fluent coryza, very often, or almost constantly, also in some cases uninterruptedly.

He cannot take cold, even though there have been strong premonitory symptoms of it, simultaneously with other great ailments from the itch malady.

Hoarseness, after the least amount of speaking; she must vomit in order to clear her voice.

Hoarseness, also sometimes aphony (she cannot speak loud but must whisper), after a slight cold.

Constant hoarseness and aphony for years; he cannot speak a loud word.

Suppuration of the larynx and the bronchia (laryngo-bronchial phthisis).[1]

Hoarseness and catarrh very often, or almost constantly; his chest is continually affected.

---

pain in the uterus and pressure toward the vagina as if everything were about to fall out, also at times most keen pains in the small of the back; the flatus is obstructed, causing pain, etc. Has the so-called uterine cancer any other origin than this (Psora) malady?

[1] Inflammation of the larynx (croup) cannot take place with any child that is free from latent Psora or has been made free from it by treatment.

Cough; frequent irritation and crawling in the throat; the cough torments him, until perspiration breaks out on his face (and on his hands).

Cough, which does not abate until there is retching and vomiting, mostly in the morning or in the evening.

Cough, which terminates every time with sneezing.

Cough mostly in the evening after lying down and whenever the head lies low.

Cough, waking the patient up after the first brief sleep.

Cough, especially in the night.

Cough, worse after awaking in the morning.

Cough, worse after eating.

Cough, at once with every deep breath.

Cough, causing a sensation of soreness in the chest, or at times stitches in the side of the chest or the abdomen.

Dry cough.

Cough; with yellow expectoration resembling pus, with or without spitting of blood.[1]

Cough, with excessive expectoration of mucus and sinking of the strength (mucous phthisis).

Attacks of whooping cough.[2]

---

[1] Suppurative pulmonary phthisis has probably seldom any other cause than this malady, even when it seems as if the fumes of quicksilver or arsenic had caused it; at least most of these cases of suppurative phthisis originate in pneumonias mismanaged with blood-letting, and this disease may always be considered as the manifestation of latent Psora.

[2] She is suddenly compelled to cough, but cannot do so, as her breath fails her, even to suffocation, with a dark-red, bloated face; usually the œsophagus is then also constricted, so that not a drop

Violent, at times unbearable, stitches in the chest at every breath ; cough impossible for pain ; without inflammatory fever (spurious pleurisy).

Pain in the chest on walking, as if the chest was about to burst.

Pressive pain in the chest, at deep breathing or at sneezing.

Often a slightly constrictive pain in the chest, which, when it does not quickly pass, causes the deepest dejection.[1]

Burning pain in the chest.

Frequent stitches in the chest, with or without cough.

Violent stitches in the side ; with great heat of the body, it is almost impossible to breathe, on account of stitches in the chest with hemoptysis and headache ; he is confined to his bed.

Night-mare ; he usually suddenly awakes at night from a frightful dream, but cannot move, nor call, nor speak, and when he endeavors to move, he suffers intolerable pains, as if he were being torn to pieces.[2]

Obstruction of the breath, with stitching pains in the chest at the slightest amount of walking ;[3] he cannot go a step farther (angina pectoris).

Asthma, merely when moving the arms, not while walking.

---

of water will pass; after eight or ten minutes, there follow eructations from the stomach, and the spasm terminates.

[1] Usually the attacks last from evening to morning, the whole night.

[2] Such attacks, in some cases, also occur several times in one night, especially when he has not been in the open air during the day.

[3] Especially when ascending a height.

Attacks of suffocation especially after midnight; the patient has to sit up, sometimes he has to leave his bed, stand stooping forward, leaning on his hands; he has to open the windows, or go out into the open air, etc.; he has palpitations; these are followed by eructations or yawning, and the spasm terminates with or without coughing and expectoration.

Palpitation with anxiety, especially at night.

Asthma, loud, difficult, at times also sibilant respiration.

Shortness of breath.

Asthma, on moving, with or without cough.

Asthma, mostly while sitting down.

Asthma, spasmodic; when she comes into the open air it takes her breath.

Asthma, in attacks, lasting several weeks.

Dwindling of the breasts, or excessive enlargement of the same, with retroceding nipples.

Erysipelas on one of the breasts (especially while nursing).

A hard, enlarging and indurating gland with lancinating pains in one of the mammæ.[1]

Itching, also moist and scaly eruptions around the nipples.

In the small of the back, in the back and in the nape of the neck, drawing (tearing), tensive pains.

Lancinating, cutting, painful stiffness of the nape of the neck; of the small of the back.

Pressive pain between the shoulder-blades.

Sensation of pressure upon the shoulders.

---

[1] Is it probable that the different varieties of cancer of the breast have any other origin than this Psora malady?

In the limbs, drawing (tearing), tensive pains, partly in the muscles and partly in the joints (rheumatism).

In the periosteum, here and there, especially in the periosteum of the long bones, pressive and pressive-drawing pains.[1]

Stitching pains in the fingers and toes.[2]

Stitches in the heels and soles of the feet while standing.

Burning in the soles of the feet.[3]

In the joints a sort of tearing, like scraping on the bone, with a red, hot swelling which is painfully sensitive to the touch and to the air, with unbearably sensitive, peevish disposition (gout, podagra, chiragra, gout in the knees, etc.).[4]

The joints of the fingers, swollen with pressive pains, painful when touching and bending them.

Thickening of the joints; they remain hard swollen, and there is pain on bending them.

The joints, as it were, stiff, with painful, difficult motion, the ligaments seem too short.[5]

Joints, painful on motion.[6]

---

[1] These spots then also pain on being touched, as if they were bruised or sore.

[2] In worse, chronic cases, this is aggravated into a cutting pain.

[3] Especially at night under a feather bed.

[4] The pains are either worse in daytime, or at night. After every attack, and when the inflammation is past, the joints of the hand are painful, as also those of the knee, the foot, those of the big toe when moved, when he stands up, etc., they feel intolerably benumbed and the limb is weakened.

[5] *E. g.*, the *lendo Achillis* on standing erect, stiffness of the tarsus, of the knees, either transient (after sitting, when rising), or permanent (contraction).

[6] *E. g.*, the shoulder-joint on raising the arm; the tarsus pains on treading as if it was about to break.

Joints crack on moving, or they make a snapping noise.

The joints are easily sprained or strained.[1]

Increasing disposition to *strains* and to *overlift* oneself even at a very slight exertion of the muscles, even in slight mechanical work, in reaching out or stretching for something high up, in lifting things that are not heavy, in quick turns of the body, pushing, etc. Such a tension or stretching of the muscles often then occasion long confinement to the bed, swoons, all grades of hysterical troubles,[2] fever, hemoptysis, etc., while persons who are not Psoric lift such burdens as their muscles are able to, without the slightest after effects.[3]

The joints are easily sprained at any false movement.[4]

---

[1] *E. g.*, the tarsus, the wrist-joint, the joint of the thumb.

[2] Often also, at once severe headache in the crown of the head, which is then also painful externally when touched, or suddenly a pain in the small of the back, or pain in the uterus, not unfrequently stitches in the side of the breast, or between the shoulder blades, which check the respiration, or painful stiffness of the neck or spine, frequently audible eructations, etc.

[3] The common people, especially in the country, seek alleviation through a sort of mesmeric stroking, but without lasting effects; the tendency to overlifting nevertheless remains. It is usually a woman (called a *stroking woman*) who makes with the tips of her thumbs passes over the shoulder blades toward the shoulders or along the spine, sometimes also from the pit of the stomach along below the ribs, only they usually exert too strong a pressure while stroking.

[4] *E. g.*, the ankle at a false step, so also the shoulder-joint. Of this kind is also the gradual luxation of the hip-joint (*i. e.*, of the head of the femur from the *acetabulum*, when the leg then becomes too long or too short, causing limping).

In the joint of the foot there is pain on treading, as if it would break.

Softening of the bones, curvature of the spine (deformity, hunchback), curvature of the long bones of the thighs and legs (*morbus anglicus*, rickets).

Fragility of the bones.

Painful sensitiveness of the skin, the muscles and of the periosteum on a moderate pressure.[1]

Intolerable[2] pain in the skin (or in the muscles, or in the periosteum) of some part of the body from a slight movement of the same or of a more distant part; *e. g.*, from writing there arises a pain in the shoulder or in the side of the neck, etc., while sawing or performing other hard labor with the same hand causes no pain; a similar pain in the adjacent parts, from speaking and moving the mouth; pain in the lips and in the back at slight touch.

Numbness of the skin or the muscles of certain parts and limbs.[3]

---

[1] As when he moderately strikes against something, it becomes very painful and for a long time; the parts on which he lies in bed are very painful, wherefore he frequently turns over at night; the posterior muscles of the thigh and the bone on which he sits are quite sore; a slight stroke with the hand on the thighs causes great pain. A slight knock against a hard object leaves blue marks, suffusion of blood.

[2] Of incredible variety. Often burning, jerking, lancinating, but often indescribable, are these pains which communicate a similar intolerable excessive sensitiveness to the mind. These pains thus affect chiefly the upper parts of the body, or the face (*tic douloureux*), or the skin of the neck, etc , at even a gentle touch, in speaking and chewing—in the shoulder at a slight pressure, or movement of the finger.

[3] The sense of touch is lacking; the parts feel hard and tumid, either periodically or permanently (constant insensibility).

Dying off of certain fingers or of the hands or feet.[1]

Crawling or also prickling formication (as from limbs going to sleep) in the arms, in the legs and in other parts (even in the finger-tips).

A crawling, or whirling, or an internally itching *restlessness*, especially in the lower limbs (in the evening in bed or early on awaking); they must be brought into another position every moment.

Painful sensation of cold in various parts.

Burning pains in various parts (frequently without any change in the usual external bodily temperature).

Coldness, repeated or constant of the whole body, or of the one side of the body; so also of single parts, cold hands, cold feet which frequently will not get warm in bed.

Chilliness, constant, even without any change in the external bodily temperature.

Frequent flushes of heat, especially in the face, more frequently with redness than without; sudden, violent sensation of heat during rest, or in slight motion, sometimes even from speaking, with or without perspiration breaking out.

Warm air in the room or at church is exceedingly repugnant to her, makes her restless, causes her to move about (at times with a pressure in the head, over the eyes, not infrequently alleviated by epistaxis).

Rushes of blood, also at times a sensation of throbbing in all the arteries (while he often looks quite pale, with a feeling of prostration throughout the body).

---

[1] The limb then becomes white, bloodless, without feeling and quite cold, often for hours, especially while it is cool (stroking with a piece of zinc toward the tips of the fingers or the toes usually drives it away quickly, but only as a palliative).

Rush of blood to the head.

Rush of blood to the chest.

Varices, varicose veins in the lower limbs (varices on the pudenda), also on the arms (even with men), often with tearing pains in them (during storms), or with itching in the varices.[1]

Erysipelas, partly in the face (with fever), partly on the limbs, on the breast while nursing, especially in a sore place (with a pricking and burning pain).

Whitlow, paronychia (sore finger with festering skin).

Chilblains (even when it is not winter) on the toes and fingers, itching, burning and lancinating pains.

Corns, which even without external pressure cause burning, lancinating pains.

Boils (furuncles), returning from time to time, especially on the nates, the thighs, the upper arms and the body. Touching them causes fine stitches in them.

Ulcers on the thighs, especially, also upon the ankles and above them and on the lower part of the calves, with itching, gnawing, tickling around the borders, and a gnawing pain as from salt on the base of the ulcer itself; the parts surrounding are of brown and bluish color, with varices near the ulcers, which, during storms and rains, often cause tearing pains, especially at night, often accompanied with erysipelas after vexation or fright, or attended with cramps in the calves.

Tumefaction and suppuration of the humerus, the femur, the patella, also of the bones of the fingers and toes (*spina ventosa*).

---

[1] The swellings of the arteries (aneurismata) seem to have no other origin than the *Psora*.

Thickening and stiffening of the joints.

Eruptions, either arising from time to time and passing away again; some voluptuously itching pustules, especially on the fingers or other parts, which, after scratching, burn and have the greatest similarity to the original itch-eruption;

or *nettlerash*, like stings and water-blisters, mostly with burning pain;

or *pimples* without pain in the face, the chest, the back, the arms and the thighs;

or *herpes* in fine miliary grains closely pressed together into round, larger or smaller spots of mostly reddish color, sometimes dry, sometimes moist, with itching, similar to the eruption of itch and with burning after rubbing them. They continually extend further to the circumference, with redness, while the middle seems to become free from the eruption and covered with smooth, shining skin (*herpes circinatus*). The moist herpes on the legs are called salt-rheum;

or *crusts* raised above the surrounding skin, round in form, with deep-red, painless borders, with frequent violent stitches on the parts of the skin not yet affected;

or *small, round spots* on the skin, covered with bran-like, dry scales, which often peel off and are again renewed without sensation;

or *red spots of the skin*, which feel dry, with burning pain; somewhat raised above the rest of the skin.

Freckles, small and round, brown or brownish spots in the face, on the hands and on the chest, without sensation.

Liver spots, large brownish spots which often cover whole limbs, the arms, the neck, the chest, etc., without sensation or with itching.

Yellowness of the skin, yellow spots of a like nature around the eyes, the mouth, on the neck, etc., without sensibility.[1]

Warts on the face, the lower arm, the hands, etc.[2]

Encysted tumors in the skin, the cellular tissue beneath it, or in the *bursæ mucosæ* of the tendons (exostosis), of various forms and sizes, cold without sensibility.[3]

Glandular swellings around the neck, in the groin, in the bend of the joints, the bend of the elbow, of the knee, in the axillæ,[4] also in the breasts.

Dryness of the (scarf) skin either on the whole body with inability to perspire through motion and heat, or only in some parts.[5]

---

[1] After riding in a carriage, yellowness of the skin comes on most quickly, if it is not yet constant but only occasional.

[2] Especially in youth. Many remain only a short time and pass away to give place to another symptom of Psora.

[3] The fungus hematodes, which has lately become such a dreadful plague, has, according to the conclusions I am compelled to draw from several cases, no other source than Psora.

[4] At times they pass over, after lancinating pains, into a sort of chronic suppuration, in which, however, instead of pus, only a colorless mucus is secreted.

[5] Especially in the hands, the outer side of the arms and legs, and even in the face; the skin is dry, rough, parched, feels chapped, and often has scales like bran.

Disagreeable sensation of dryness over the whole body (also in the face, around and in the mouth, in the throat, or in the nose, although the breath passes freely through it).

Perspiration comes too easily from slight motion; even while sitting, he is attacked with perspiration all over, or merely on some parts; *e. g.*, almost constant perspiration of the hands and feet,[1] so also strong perspiration in the axillæ[2] and around the pudenda.

Daily morning sweats, often causing the patient to drip, this for many years, often with sour or pungent-sour smell.[3]

One-sided perspiration, only on one side of the body, or only on the upper part of the body, or only on the lower part.

Increasing susceptibility to colds, either of the whole body (often even from repeatedly wetting the hands, now with warm water, then with cold, as in washing clothes), or only susceptibility of certain parts of the body, of the head, the neck, the chest, the abdomen, the feet, etc., often in a moderate or slight draught, or after slightly moistening these parts;[4] even from

---

[1] The latter is usually very fetid and so abundant that, after even a short walk, the soles of the feet, the heels and toes are soaked and sore.

[2] Not infrequently of red color or of a rank smell like that of he goats or that of garlic.

[3] Here belongs the perspiration of Psoric children on their head after going to sleep in the evening.

[4] The ailments following from it, immediately afterwards, are then considerable and manifold: Pains in the limbs, headaches, catarrh, sore throat, and inflammation of the throat, coryza, swelling of the glands of the neck, hoarseness, cough, dyspnœa, stitches

being in a cooler room, in a rainy atmosphere, or with a low barometer.

So-called *weather prophets*, *i. e.*, renewed severe pains in parts of the body which were formerly injured, wounded, or broken, though they have since been healed and cicatrized; this renewed pain sets in, when great changes of the weather, great cold, or a storm are imminent, or when a thunder storm is in the air.

Watery swelling, either of the feet alone, or in one foot, or in the hands, or the face, or the abdomen, or the scrotum, etc., alone, or again cutaneous swelling over the whole body (dropsies).

Attacks of sudden heaviness of the arms and legs.

Attacks of paralytic weakness and paralytic lassitude of the one arm, the one hand, the one leg, without pain, either arising suddenly and passing quickly, or commencing gradually and constantly increasing.

Sudden bending of the knee.

Children fall easily, without any visible cause. Also similar attacks of weakness, with adults, in the legs, so that in walking one foot glides this way and the other that way, etc.

While walking in the open air sudden attacks of faintness, especially in the legs.[1]

---

in the chest, fever, troubles of digestion, colic, vomiting, diarrhœa, stomachache, rising of water from the stomach, also stitches in the face and other parts, jaundice-like color of the skin, etc. No person who is not Psoric ever suffers the least after-effects from such causes.

[1] At times the feeling of faintness seems to rise up even to the scrobiculus cordis, where it turns into a ravenous hunger, which suddenly deprives him of all strength; he is attacked with tremor and has immediately to lie down for a while.

While sitting, the patient feels intolerably weary, but stronger while walking.

The predisposition to spraining and straining the joints at a mis-step, or a wrong grasp, increases at times even to dislocation, *e. g.*, in the tarsus, the shoulder-joint, etc.

The snapping and cracking of the joints at any motion of the limb increases with a disagreeable sensation.

The going to sleep of the limbs increases and follows on slight causes, *e. g.*, in supporting the head with the arm, crossing the legs while sitting, etc.

The painful cramps in some of the muscles increase and come on without appreciable cause.

Slow, spasmodic straining of the flexor muscles of the limbs.

Sudden jerks of some muscles and limbs even while waking; *e. g.*, of the tongue, the lips, the muscles of the face, of the pharynx, of the eyes, of the jaws, of the hands and of the feet.

Tonic shortening of the flexor muscles (tetanus).

Involuntary turning and twisting of the head, or the limbs, with full consciousness (St. Vitus' dance).

Sudden fainting spells and sinking of the strength, with loss of consciousness.

Attacks of tremor in the limbs, without anxiety. Continuous, constant trembling, also in some cases beating with the hands, the arms, the legs.

Attacks of loss of consciousness, lasting a moment or a minute, with an inclination of the head to the one shoulder, with or without jerks of one part or the other.

Epilepsies of various kinds.

Almost constant yawning, stretching and straining of the limbs.

Sleepiness during the day, often immediately after sitting down, especially after meals.

Difficulty in falling asleep, when abed in the evening; he often lies awake for hours.

He passes the nights in a mere slumber.

Sleeplessness, from anxious heat, every night, an anxiety which sometimes rises so high, that he must get up from his bed and walk about.

After three o'clock in the morning, no sleep, or at least no sound sleep.

As soon as he closes his eyes, all manner of phantastic appearances and distorted faces appear.

In going to sleep, she is disquieted by strange, anxious fancies; she has to get up and walk about.

Very vivid dreams, as if awake; or sad, frightful, anxious, vexing, lascivious dreams.

Loud talking, screaming, during sleep.

Somnambulism; he rises up at night, while sleeping with closed eyes, and attends to various duties; he performs even dangerous feats with ease, without knowing anything about them when awake.

Attacks of suffocation while sleeping (nightmare).

Various sorts of severe pains at night, or nocturnal thirst, dryness of the throat, of the mouth, or frequent urinating at night.

Early on awaking, dizzy, indolent, unrefreshed, as if he had not done sleeping and more tired than in the evening, when he lay down; it takes him several hours (and only after rising) before he can recover from this weariness.

After a very restless night, he often has more strength in the morning, than after a quiet, sound sleep.

Intermittent fever, even when there are no cases about, either sporadic or epidemic,[1] or endemic; the form, duration and type of the fever are very various; quotidian, tertian, quartan, quintan or every seven days.

Every evening, chills with blue nails.

Every evening, single chills.

Every evening, heat, with a rush of blood to the head, with red cheeks, also at times an intervening chill.

Intermittent fever of several weeks' duration, followed by a moist itching eruption lasting several weeks, but which is healed again during a like period of intermittent fever, and alternating thus for years.

Disturbances of the mind and spirit of all kinds.[2]

Melancholy by itself, or with insanity, also at times alternating with frenzy and hours of rationality.

Anxious oppression, early on awaking.

Anxious oppression in the evening after going to bed.[3]

---

[1] Epidemic intermittent fevers probably never seize a man who is free from Psora, so that wherever there is a susceptibility to them, it is to be accounted a symptom of Psora.

[2] I have never either in my practice, nor in any insane asylum, seen a patient suffering from melancholy, insanity, or frenzy whose disease did not have *Psora* as its foundation, complicated at times, however, though rarely, with syphilis.

[3] This causes some patients to break out into a strong perspiration; others feel from it merely flushes of blood and throbbing in all the arteries; with others, the anxious oppression tends to constrict

Anxiety, several times a day (with and without pains), or at certain hours of the day or of the night; usually the patient then finds no rest, but has to run hither and thither, and often falls into perspiration.

Melancholy, palpitation and anxiousness causes her at night to wake up from sleep (mostly just before the beginning of the menses).

Mania of self-destruction[1] (spleen?).

---

the throat, threatening suffocation, while others have a sensation, as if all the blood in their arteries were standing still, causing anguish. With others, this oppression is associated with anxious images and thoughts, and seems to rise from them, while with others, there is oppression without anxious ideas and thoughts.

[1] This kind of disease of the mind or spirit, which is also merely psoric, seems not to have been taken into consideration. Without feeling any anxiety, or anxious thoughts, therefore, also, without any one's perceiving such anxiety in them, apparently in the full exercise of their reason, they are impelled, urged, yea, compelled by a certain feeling of necessity, to self-destruction. They are only healed by a cure of *Psora*, if their utterances are noticed *in time*. I say *in time*, for in the last stages of this kind of insanity it is peculiarly characteristic of this disease, not to utter anything about such a determination to anyone. This frenzy manifests itself in fits of one-half or of whole hours, usually in the end daily, often at certain times of the day. But besides these fits of destructive mania, such persons have usually also fits of anxious oppression, which seem, however, to be independent of the former fits, and come at other hours, accompanied partly with pulsation in the pit of the stomach, but during these they are not tormented with the desire of taking their own life. These attacks of anxiety which seem to be more of a bodily nature, and are not connected with the other train of thoughts, may also be lacking, while the fits of suicidal mania rule in a high degree; they may also return, when that mania is in a great part extinguished through the antipsoric remedies, so that the two seem to be independent of one another, though they have the same original malady for their foundation.

A weeping mood; they often weep for hours without knowing a cause for it.[1]

Attacks of fear; *e. g.*, fear of fire, of being alone, of apoplexy, of becoming insane, etc.

Attacks of passion, resembling frenzy.

Fright caused by the merest trifles; this often causes perspiration and trembling.

Disinclination to work, in persons who else are most industrious; no impulse to occupy himself, but rather the most decided repugnance thereto.[2]

Excessive sensitiveness.[3]

Irritability from weakness.[3]

---

[1] This is a symptom, however, which seems to be caused by the diseased state, especially of the female sex, in order to soothe temporarily more and greater nervous disorders.

[2] Such a person, when she desired to begin one of her domestic occupations, was seized with anxiety and oppression; her limbs trembled, and she became suddenly so weary, she had to lie down.

[3] All physical and psychical impressions, even the weaker and the weakest, cause a morbid excitement, often in a high degree. Occurrences affecting the mind, not only such as are of sad and vexatious kind, but also those of a joyous kind, cause surprising ailments and disorders; touching tales, yea, even thinking of them and recalling them, cause a tumultuous excitement of the nerves, and drive the anxiety into the head, etc. Even a little reading about indifferent things, or looking attentively at an object; *e. g.*, while sewing, attentively listening even to indifferent things, too bright a light, the loud talking of several people at the same time, even single tones on a musical instrument, the ringing of bells, etc., cause harmful impressions: trembling, weariness, headache, chills, etc. Often the senses of smell and taste are immoderately sensitive. In many cases even moderate bodily motion, or speaking, also moderate warmth, cold, open air, wetting the skin with water, etc. Not a few suffer even in their room from a sudden change in the weather, while most of these patients complain dur-

Quick change of moods; often very merry and exuberantly so, often again and, indeed, very suddenly, dejection; *e. g.*, on account of his disease, or from other trifling causes. Sudden transition from cheerfulness to sadness, or vexation without a cause.

These are some of the leading symptoms observed by me, which, if they are often repeated, or become constant, show that the internal *Psora* is coming forth from its latent state. They are at the same time the elements, from which (under unfavorable external conditions) the itch-malady, as it manifests itself, composes the illimitable number of chronic diseases, and with one man assumes the one form, with another another, according to the bodily constitution, defects in the education, habits, employment and external circumstances, as also modified by the various psychical and physical impressions. It thus unfolds into manifold forms of disease, with so many varieties, that they are by no means exhausted by the disease-symptoms enumerated in the pathology of the old-school, and erroneously designated there as well-defined, constant and peculiar diseases.*

---

ing stormy and wet weather, few of dry weather with a clear sky The full moon also with some persons, and the new moon with others, has an unfavorable effect.

*They bear the following names: Scrofula, rickets, spina ventosa, atrophy, marasmus, consumption, pulmonary consumption ,asthma, tabes mucosa, laryngeal phthisis, chronic catarrh, constant coryza, difficult dentition, worms and consequent diseases, dyspepsia, abdomina, cramps, hypochondria, hysteria, dropsy, dropsy of the abdomenl dropsy of the ovaries, of the uterus, hydrocele, hydrocephalus, amenorrhœa, dysmenorrhœa, uterine hemorrhages, hematemesis, hemoptysis and hemorrhages, vaginal hemorrhages, dysuria,

These are the characteristic secondary symptoms* of the long-unacknowledged, thousand-headed monster, pregnant with disease, the *Psora*, the original miasmatic malady which now makes its manifest appearance.†

---

ischuria, enuresis, diabetes, catarrh of the bladder, hematuria, nephralgia, gravel of the kidneys, stricture of the urethra, stricture of the intestines, blind and running piles, fistula of the rectum, difficult stools, constipation, chronic diarrhœa, induration of the liver, jaundice, cyanosis, heart diseases, palpitation, spasms of the chest, dropsy of the chest, abortion, sterility, metromania, impotence, induration of the testicles, dwindling of the testicles, prolapsus uteri, inversion of the womb, inguinal, femoral and umbilical hernias, dislocations of the joints from an internal cause, curvature of the spine, chronic inflammation of the eyes, fistula lachrymalis, short-sightedness and long-sightedness, day blindness and night blindness, obscuration of the cornea, cataracts, glaucoma, amaurosis, deafness, deficient smell or taste, chronic one-sided headache, megrim, tic douloureux, tinea capitis, scab, crusta lactea, tetters (herpes), pimples, nettlerash, encysted tumors, goitre, varices, aneurism, erysipelas, sarcomas, osteosarcoma, scirrhus, cancer of the lips, cheeks, breast, uterus, fungus hematodes, rheumatism, gout in the hips, knotty gout, podagra, apoplectic fits, swoons, vertigo, paralysis, contractions, tetanus, convulsions, epilepsy, St. Vitus' dance, melancholy, insanity, imbecility, nervous debility, etc.

*The supreme royal councillor *Kopp*, an Allopath, who is unwillingly and only half and half approaching Homœopathy, pretends to have seen chronic diseases disappear of themselves—he may have seen some particular symptoms disappear, which symptoms the old school, in its shortsighted fashion, considered with him as so many entire diseases!

†I will grant that the doctrine, that "all chronic non-venereal diseases which are not extinguishable by the vital force, in an orderly course of life, while external circumstances are favorable, but which even increase with the years, are of psoric origin," is for

all who have not fully weighed my reasons and for all narrow-minded people, too great, too overwhelming. But it is none the less true. Or should we regard such a chronic disease as not being psoric, because the patient cannot remember that he at some-time, all the way back to his birth, has had several or more (intolerable voluptuously) itching pustules of itch on his skin, or (since the itch-disease is considered as something disgraceful) is not willing to acknowledge it? His non-acknowledgment here proves nothing to the contrary.

Since at all times, all the innumerable chronic diseases resulting from an acknowledged preceding itch (when this has not been cured) are ineradicable through the vital force, and advance in their equable course as psoric ailments, and continually aggravated; so long as the doubters of the psora doctrine cannot show me *any other source* which is at least as probable for a (non-veneric) ailment, which, despite of favorable external conditions, correct diet, good morality and vigorous bodily constitution, nevertheless increases every year, without any preceding infection from itch so far as memory goes; so long as I have on my side an overpowering analogous probability, *i. e.*, 100 to 1, that also the individual cases of chronic disease, which show *a like progression*, probably also are, yea, must be of a psoric nature, although the patient cannot or will not remember a preceding infection.

It is easy to doubt matters which cannot be laid before our ocular vision, but in itself this doubt proves nothing at all, for according to the old rule of logic: *negantis est probare.*

To prove the Psoric nature of these chronic diseases without acknowledged infection, we do not even need the fact that the anti-psoric remedies prove effectual therein; this serves only like the proof to a correctly solved mathematical problem.

Now since, in addition, the other remedies, although also selected according to the similarity of their symptoms, do not by far yield so durable and thorough a cure in such chronic diseases, as those which are recognized as anti-psoric, and which are selected in as Homœopathic a manner, because these more than the others are adequate to the whole extent of the endless number of symptoms of the great Psora malady: I do not see why men will deny to the latter the title of the especially *anti-psoric* remedies, unless this springs from dogmatism.

And just as little is there any good reason for contradicting me, when I (*Organon*, § 73) explain the acute diseases which return from time to time; *e. g.*, inflammations of the throat, of the chest, etc., as flaming up from a latent *Psora*, simply because their inflammatory state, as they say, is mostly to be combatted by means of the anti-phlogistic remedies, which are not anti-psoric; *i. e.*, Aconite, Belladonna, Mercury and the like. These, nevertheless, have their source in a latent Psora, because their customary return cannot be prevented by anything but a final cure with anti-psoric remedies.

Cure of the Chronic Diseases.

CURE.

We now proceed to the medical Homœopathic treatment of the illimitably large number of chronic diseases, which, after the above gained knowledge of their threefold nature, has not, indeed, become easy, but—what without this knowledge was before impossible—has at last become *possible*, since the homœpathically specific remedies for each one of these three different miasmata have in great part been discovered.

The first two miasmata, which cause by far the smaller part of the chronic diseases, the *venereal chancre-disease* (syphilis) and the *figwart-disease* (sycosis), with their sequelæ, we will treat first, in order that we may have a free path to the therapeutics of the immeasurably greater number of the various chronic diseases which spring from *Psora*.

SYCOSIS.

First, then, concerning sycosis, as being that miasma which has produced by far the fewest chronic diseases, and has only been dominant from time to time. This *fig-wart disease*, which in later times, especially during the French war, in the years 1809–1814, was so widely spread, but which has since showed itself more and more rarely, was treated, almost always, in an inefficient and injurious manner, internally with Mercury, because it was considered homogeneous with the venereal chancre-disease; but the excrescences on the genitals were treated by Allopathic physicians always in the most violent external way by cauterizing, burning and cutting, or by ligatures. These excrescences usually first manifest themselves on the genitals, and appear usually, but not always, attended with a sort of gonorrhœa* from the urethra, several days or several weeks, even many weeks after infection through coition; more rarely they appear dry and like warts, more frequently soft, spongy, emitting a specifically fetid fluid (sweetish and almost like herring-brine),

---

*Usually in gonorrhœa of this kind, the discharge is from the beginning thickish, like pus; micturition is less difficult, but the body of the penis swollen somewhat hard; the penis is also in some cases covered on the back with glandular tubercles, and very painful to the touch.

bleeding easily, and in the form of a coxcomb or a cauliflower (*brassica botrytes*). These, with males, sprout forth on the glans and on, or below, the prepuce, but with women, on the parts surrounding the pudenda; and the pudenda themselves, which are then swollen, are covered often by a great number of them. When these are violently removed, the natural, proximate effect is, that they will usually come forth again, usually to be subjected again, in vain, to a similar, painful, cruel treatment. But even if they could be rooted out in this way, it would merely have the consequence, that the fig-wart disease, after having been deprived of the local symptom which acts vicariously for the internal ailment, would appear* in other and much worse ways, in secondary ailments; for the fig-wart miasm, which rules in the whole organism, has been in no way diminished, either by the external destruction of the above-mentioned excrescences, or by the Mercury which has been used internally, and which is in no way appropriate to sycosis. Besides the undermining of the general health by Mercury, which in this disease can only do

---

*The miasm of the other common gonorrhœa seems not to penetrate the whole organism, but only to locally stimulate the urinary organs. They yield either to a dose of one drop of fresh parsley-juice, when this is indicated by a frequent urgency to urinate, or a small dose of Cannabis, of Cantharides, or of the Copaiva balm, according to their different constitution and the other ailments attending it. These should, however, be always used in the higher and highest dynamizations (potencies), unless a Psora, slumbering in the body of the patient, has been developed by means of a strongly affecting, irritating or weakening treatment by Allopathic physicians. In such a case frequently secondary gonorrhœas remain, which can only be cured by an anti-psoric treatment.

injury, and which is given mostly in very large doses and in the most active preparations, similar excrescences then break out in other parts of the body, either whitish, spongy, sensitive, flat elevations, in the cavity of the mouth, on the tongue, the palate and the lips, or as large, raised, brown and dry tubercles in the axillæ, on the neck, on the scalp, etc., or there arise other ailments of the body, of which I shall only mention the contraction of the tendons of the flexor muscles, especially of the fingers.

The gonorrhœa dependent on the fig-wart miasma, as well as the above-mentioned excrescences (*i. e.*, the whole sycosis), are cured most surely and most thoroughly through the internal use of Thuja,* which, in this case, is Homœopathic, in a dose of a few pellets as large as poppy seeds, moistened with the dilution potentized to the decillionth† degree, and when these have exhausted their action after fifteen, twenty, thirty, forty days, alternating with just as small a dose of Nitric acid, diluted to the decillionth degree, which must be allowed to act as long a time, in order to remove the gonorrhœa and the excrescences; *i. e.*, the whole sycosis. It is not necessary to use any external application, except in *the most inveterate and difficult* cases, when the larger fig-warts may be moistened every day with the mild, pure juice pressed from the green leaves of Thuja, mixed with an equal quantity of Alcohol.

---

*Materia Medica Pura, Part V.

†If further doses of Thuja are required, they are used most efficiently from other potencies (viii., vi., v., ii.), a change of the modification of the remedy, which facilitates and strengthens its ablity of affecting the vital force.

But if the patient was at the same time affected with another chronic ailment, as if usual after the violent treatment of fig-warts by Allopathic physicians, then we often find developed Psora* complicated with sycosis, when the Psora, as is often the case, was latent before in the patient. At times, when a badly treated case of venereal chancre disease had preceded, both these miasmata are conjoined in a three-fold complication with syphilis. Then it is necessary first to come to the assistance of the most afflicted part, the *Psora*, with the specific anti-psoric remedies given below, and then to make use of the remedies for sycosis, before the proper dose of the best preparation of Mercury, as will be described below, is given against the syphilis; the same alternating treatment may be continued, until a complete cure is effected. Only, each one of these three kinds of medicine must be given the proper time to complete its action.

In this reliable cure of sycosis from within, no external remedy (except the juice of Thuja in inveterate bad cases) must be applied or laid on the fig-warts, only clean, dry lint, if they are of the moist variety.

---

*This Psora is hardly ever found in its developed state (and thus capable of entering into complication with other miasmata) with young people who have just been infected and seized by the fig-wart disease, and who have not had to pass through the usual Mercurial treatment, which never runs its course without the most violent assaults on the constitution; by this pernicious derangement of the whole organism, the Psora, even if slumbering ever so soundly, will be awakened, if as is often the case, it was present within.

SYPHILIS.

The second chronic miasma, which is more widely spread than the figwart-disease, and which for three and a half [now four] centuries has been the source of many other chronic ailments, is the miasm of the venereal disease proper, the chancre-disease (syphilis). This disease only causes difficulties in its cure, if it is entangled (complicated) with a Psora that has been already far developed—with sycosis it is complicated but rarely, but then usually at the same time with Psora.

In the cure of the venereal disease, three states are to be distinguished:

1. When syphilis is still alone and attended with its associated local symptom, the *chancre*, or at least if this has been removed by external applications, it is still associated with the other local symptom, which in a similar manner acts vicariously for the internal disorder, the bubo.*

2. When it is alone, indeed, *i. e.*, without any complication with a second or third miasma, but has already been deprived of the vicarious local symptom, the chancre (and the bubo).

* Very rarely the impure coition is at once followed by the bubo alone without any preceding chancre; usually the bubo only comes after the destruction of the chancre by local applications, and is a very troublesome substitute for the same.

3. When it is already complicated with another chronic disease, *i. e.*, with a Psora already developed, while the local symptom may either be yet present, or may have been removed by local applications.

The chancre appears, after an impure coition, usually between the seventh and fourteenth days, rarely sooner or later, mostly on the member infected with the miasma, first as a little pustule, which changes into an impure ulcer with raised borders and stinging pains, which if not cured remains standing on the same place during man's lifetime, only increasing with the years, while the secondary symptoms of the venereal disease, syphilis, cannot break out as long as it exists.

In order to help in such a case, the Allopathic physician destroys this chancre, by means of corroding, cauterizing and desiccating substances, wrongly conceiving it to be a sore arising merely from without through a local infection, thus holding it to be a merely local ulcer, such also it is declared to be in their writings. They falsely suppose, that when it appears, no internal venereal disease is as yet to be thought of, so that when locally exterminating the chancre, they suppose that they remove all the venereal disease from the patient at once, if only he will not permit this ulcer to remain too long in its place, so that the absorbent vessels do not get time to transfer the poison into the internal organism, and so cause by delay a general infection of the system with syphilis. They evidently do not know that the venereal infection of the whole body commenced with the very moment of the impure coition, and was already completed before the appearance of the chancre. The

Allopathic doctor destroys in his blindness, through local applications, the vicarious external symptom (the chancre ulcer), which kind nature intended for the alleviation of the internal extensive venereal general disease ; and so he inexorably compels the organism to replace the destroyed first substitute of the internal venereal malady (the chancre) by a far more painful substitute, the bubo, which hastens onward to suppuration ; and when the Allopath, as is usually the case, also drives out this bubo through his injurious treatment, then nature finds itself compelled to develop the internal malady through far more troublesome secondary ailments, through the outbreak of the whole chronic syphilis, and nature accomplishes this, though slowly (frequently not before several months have elapsed), but with *unfailing certainty*. Instead of assisting, therefore, the Allopath does injury.

John Hunter says:* "Not one patient out of fifteen will escape syphilis, if the chancre is destroyed by mere external applications," and in another passage in his book† he says: "The result of destroying the chancre ever so early, and even on the first day of its appearance, if this is effected by local applications, was always the consequent outbreak of syphilis."

Just as emphatically Fabre declares:‡ "Syphilis always follows on the destruction of the chancre by local applications. He relates that *Petit* cut off a part

* *Abhandl. über die vener. Krankheit* (Treatise on the Venereal Disease), Leipsic, 1787, p. 531.

† *Abhandl. über die vener. Krankheit*, Leipsic, 1787, pp. 551–553.

‡ *Fabre, Lettres, Supplément à son traité des maladies* vénériennes. *Paris*, 1786.

of the labia of a woman, who had thereon for a few days a venereal chancre; the wound healed, but syphilis, nevertheless, broke out."

How, then, could physicians, despite all these facts and testimonies, close their eyes and ears to the truth: that the whole venereal disease (syphilis) was already developed within, before the chancre could appear, and that it was a most unpardonable mistake to forward the certain outbreak of the syphilis, already present within, into the venereal disease, by driving away and destroying the chancre by external means, and thereby destroying the fair opportunity afforded of curing this disease in the easiest and most convincing manner, through the internal specific remedy, while the chancre was yet fully present! The disease is not cured except when through the effect of the internal remedy alone, the chancre is cured; but it is fully extinguished, as soon as through the action of the internally operating medicine alone (without the addition of any external remedy) the chancre is completely cured, without leaving any trace of its former presence.

I have never, in my practice of more than fifty years, seen any trace of the venereal disease break out, so long as the chancre remained untouched in its place, even if this were a space of several years (for it never passes away of itself), and even when it had largely increased in its place, as is natural in time with the internal augmentation of the venereal disorder, which increase takes place in time in every chronic miasma.

But whenever anyone is so imprudent, as to destroy

this vicarious local symptom, the organism is ready to cause the internal syphilis to break out into the venereal disease, since the general venereal disease dwells in the body from the first moment of infection.

For in the spot, into which at the impure coition the syphilitic miasma had been first rubbed in and had been caught, it is, in the same moment, no more local; the whole living body has already received (perceived) its presence, the miasma has already become the property of the whole organism. All wiping off and washing off, however speedy, and with whatever fluid this be done (and as we have seen, even with the exsection of the part affected), it is too late—is in vain. There is not to be perceived, indeed, any morbid transmutation in that spot during the first days, but the specific venereal transformation takes place in the internal of the body irresistibly, from the first moment of infection until syphilis has developed itself throughout the whole body, and only then (not before), nature loaded down by the internal malady, brings forth the local symptom peculiar to this malady, the chancre, usually in the place first infected; and this symptom is intended by nature to soothe the internal completed malady.

Therefore, also, the cure of the venereal disease is effected most easily and in the most convincing manner, so long as the chancre (the bubo) has not yet been driven out by local applications, so long as the chancre (the bubo) still remains unchanged, as a vicarious symptom of the internal syphilis. In this state, and especially when it is not yet complicated with Psora, it may be asserted from manifold experience and with good reason, *that there is on earth no chronic miasma, no chronic disease springing from a miasma, which is more curable and more easily curable than this.*

In this *first* simple state and simple cure, when the chancre (or the bubo) is still present, and there is no complication with a developed Psora, no prominent chronic ailment from a Psoric origin (usually there is none such with young, lively persons), and with latent Psora syphilis combines as little as sycosis—in this *first* state it needs only one little dose of the best mercurial remedy, in order to cure thoroughly and forever the whole syphilis with its chancre, within fourteen days. In a few days after taking such a dose of mercury, the chancre (without any external application) becomes a clean sore with a little mild pus, and heals of itself—as a convincing proof, that the venereal malady is also fully extinguished within; and it does not leave behind the least scar, or the least spot, showing any other color than the other healthy skin. But the chancre, which is not treated with external application, would never heal, if the internal syphilis had not been already annihilated and extinguished by the dose of mercury; for so long as it exists in its place, it is the natural and unmistakable proof of even the least remainder of an existing syphilis.

I have, indeed, in the second edition of the first part of *Materia Medica Pura* (Dresden, 1822), described the preparation of the pure semi-oxide of mercury, and I still consider this to be one of the most excellent anti-syphilitic medicines; but it is difficult to prepare it in sufficient purity. In order, therefore, to reach this wished for goal in a still simpler manner, free from all detours, and yet just as perfectly (for in the preparation of medicines we cannot proceed in too simple a manner), it is best to proceed in the way given below, so that one grain of quite pure running quick-silver is triturated three times, with 100 grains of sugar of milk each time, up to the millionth attenuation, in three hours, and one grain of this third trituration is dissolved, and then potentized through twenty-seven diluting phials up to (x) the decillionth degree, as is taught at the end of this volume, with respect to the dynamization of the other dry medicines.

I formerly used the billionth dynamization (ii) of this preparation in 1, 2 or 3 fine pellets moistened with this dilution, as a dose, and this was done successfully for such cures; although the preparation of the higher potencies (iv, vi, vii), and finally the decillionth potency (x), show some advantages, in their quick, penetrating and yet mild action for this purpose; but in cases where a second or third dose (however seldom needed) should be found necessary, a lower potency may then be taken.

Just as the continued presence of the chancre (or the bubo) during the cure shows the continued presence of syphilis, so when the chancre (and the bubo) heal merely from the internally applied Mercury, without any addition of a remedy used for the local symptom, and yet this disappears without leaving any trace of its former presence; it is incontrovertibly sure, that also every trace of the internal syphilis was extinguished at the moment of the completion of the cure of the chancre or the bubo.

But just as incontrovertibly does it follow that every

disappearance of the chancre (or the bubo) owing to a mere local destruction, since it was no real cure founded on the extirpation of the internal venereal disease through the internally given appropriate Mercury medicine, leaves to us the certainty that the syphilis remains behind; and every one who supposes himself healed by any such merely local, pretended cure, is to be considered as much venereally diseased as he was before the destruction of the chancre.

The *second* state in which, as mentioned above, syphilis may have to be treated, is the rare case when an otherwise healthy person, affected with no other chronic disease (and thus without any developed Psora), has experienced this injudicious driving away of the chancre through local applications, effected by an ordinary physician in a short time and without attacking the organism overmuch with internal and external remedies. Even in such a case,—as we have not as yet to combat any complication with Psora—all outbreaks of the secondary venereal disease may be avoided, and the man may be freed from every trace of the venereal miasma through the before-mentioned simple internal cure effected by a like dose of the above-mentioned Mercurial medicine although the certainty of his cure can no more be so manifestly proved as if the chancre had still been in existence during this internal cure, and as if it had become a mild ulcer simply through this internal remedy, and had been thus manifestly cured of itself.

But here also there may be found a sign of the non-completed as well as of the completed cure of the internal syphilis which has not yet broken out into the venereal disease; but this sign will only manifest itself to an exact observer. In case the chancre has been driven out through local application, even if the remedies used had not been very acrid, there will always remain in the place where it stood, as a sign of the unextinguished internal syphilis, a discolored, reddish, red or blue scar; while on the contrary when the cure of the whole venereal disease has been effected by the internal remedy, and if thus the chancre heals of itself without the action of an external application, and when it disappears because it is no more needed as a substitute and alleviator of an internal venereal disorder which now has ceased, then the spot of the former chancre can no more be recognized, for the skin covering that place will be just as smooth and of the same color as the rest, so that no trace can be discerned of the spot where the chancre had stood.

Now if the Homœopathic physician has carefully taken cognizance of the presence of the discolored scar remaining after the quick, merely local expulsion of the venereal local symptom, as a sign of the unextinguished internal syphilis, and if the person to be healed is otherwise in good health, and consequently his venereal disorder is not yet complicated with Psora, he will also, even now, be able to free him from every remainder of the venereal miasma by one dose of the best preparation of Mercury as above described, and he will be convinced that the cure is completed, from the fact that during the time of the activity of the specific remedy the scar will again assume the healthy color of the other skin and all discoloration of that spot will disappear.

Even when, after the expulsion of the chancre by local applications, the bubo has already broken out but the patient is not yet seized with any other chronic disease, and consequently the internal syphilis is not yet complicated with a developed Psora (which is nevertheless a rare case), the same treatment will also here, while the bubo is only developing, produce a cure; and its completion will be recognized by the same signs.

In both cases, if they have been rightly treated, the cure is a complete one, and no outbreak of the venereal disease need any more be apprehended.

The most difficult of all these cases, the *third*, is still to be treated: when the man at the time of the syphilitic infection was already laboring under a chronic disease, so that his syphilis was complicated with Psora, even while the chancre yet existed, or when, even while there was no chronic disease in the body at the outbreak of the chancre, and the indwelling Psora could only be recognized by its tokens, an allopathic physician has, nevertheless, destroyed the local symptom, not only slowly and with very painful external applications, but has also subjected him for a long time to an internal treatment, weakening and strongly affecting him, so that the general health has been undermined and the Psora which has as yet been latent within him has been brought to its development and has broken out into chronic ailments, and these irrepressibly combine with the internal syphilis, the local symptom of which had been at the same time destroyed in such an irrational manner. Psora can only be complicated with the venereal disease when it has been developed and when it has ultimated itself in a manifest chronic disease; but not when it is as yet latent and slumbering. By the latter the cure of syphilis is not obstructed, but *when complicated with developed Psora, it is impossible to cure the venereal disease alone.*

Only too often, I should say, do we find the syphilis which has remained uncured after the merely local destruction of the chancre, complicated with awakened Psora, not always because the Psora was already developed before the venereal infection—for this is rarely the case with young people—but because it is violently awakened and brought to its outbreak by the usual treatment of the venereal disease. By means of friction with Mercury, large doses of Calomel, Corrosive sublimate and similar acrid Mercurial remedies (which originate fever, dysenteric abdominal ailments, chronic exhausting salivation, pains in the limbs, sleeplessness, etc., without possessing sufficient anti-syphilitic power to cure the chancre-miasma mildly, quickly and perfectly), they assault the venereal patient often for many months, with the intermediate use of many weakening warm baths and purgatives; so that the internal slumbering Psora (whose nature causes it to break forth in all great convulsions and in the weakening of the general health) is awakened before the syphilis can be cured by such an injudicious treatment, and thus becomes associated and complicated therewith.

There arises in this manner and through this combination what is called a *masked, spurious syphilis*, and in England *pseudo syphilis*, a monster of a double disease,* which no physician hitherto has been able to

* Yea, after such a treatment it is even more than a double disease; the sharp Mercurial medicines, in large and frequent doses,

cure, because no physician hitherto has been acquainted with the Psora in its great extent and its nature, neither in its latent nor its developed state; and no one suspected this dreadful combination with syphilis, much less perceived it. No one, therefore, could heal the developed Psora, the only cause of the uncurableness of this bastard syphilis,—nor could they in consequence free the syphilis from this horrible combination so as to make it curable, just as the Psora remains incurable if the syphilis has not been extirpated.

In order to reach this so-called masked venereal disease successfully, the following rule must serve the homœopathic physician: After removing all hurtful influences that affect the patient from without and after settling on a light and yet nourishing and strengthening diet for the patient, let him first give the antipsoric medicine which is homœopathically the best fitting to the then prevailing state of disease, as will be shown below, and when this medicine has completed its action, also probably a second, most suitable to the still prominent Psora symptoms, and these should be allowed to act against the Psora, until they have effected all that can be at present done against it—then should be given the dose above described of the best Mercurial preparation to act against the venereal disease for three, five to seven weeks; *i. e.*, so long as it will continue to produce an improvement in the venereal symptoms.

---

have also added their medicinal disease, which when we consider in addition the debility caused by such treatment, must place the patient in a most sad state. In such a case Hepar sulphuris is probably to be preferred to the pure Sulphur.

In inveterate and difficult cases, however, this first course will hardly accomplish all that is desired. There usually still remain some ailments and disorders, which cannot be definitely classed as purely psoric, and others which cannot be classed as definitely syphilitic, and these require still some additional aid. A repetition of a similar process of cure is here required; *i. e.*, first another application of one or more of the antipsoric remedies that have not yet been used, and which are homœopathically the most appropriate, until whatever seems still unsyphilitically morbid—*i. e.*, psoric—may disappear, when the before mentioned dose of the Mercurial remedy, but in another potency, should be given again and allowed to complete its action, until the manifest venereal symptoms (the pricking, painful ulcer of the tonsils, the round copper-colored spots that shimmer through the epidermis, the eruptive pimples which do not itch and are found chiefly in the face upon a bluish-red foundation, the painless cutaneous ulcers on the scalp and the penis, which are smooth, pale, clean, merely covered with mucus, and almost level with the healthy skin, etc., and the boring nightly pains in the exostoses) have entirely passed away. But since the secondary venereal symptoms are so changeable that their temporary disappearance gives no certainty of their complete extinction, we must also wait for that more conclusive sign of the complete extirpation of the venereal miasm afforded by the return of the healthy color and the entire disappearance of the discoloration found in the scar which remains after the extirpation of the chancre by local, corrosive applications.

I have, in my practice, found only two cases* of the threefold complication of the three chronic miasms, the fig-wart disease with the venereal chancre miasm and at the same time a developed Psora, and these cases were cured according to the same method; *i. e.*, the Psora was treated first, then the one of the other two chronic miasmata, the symptoms of which were at the time the most prominent, and then the last one. The remaining psoric symptoms had then still to be combatted with suitable remedies, and then lastly what there yet remained of sycosis or syphilis, by means of the remedies given above. I would also remark that the complete cure of sycosis which has taken possession of the whole organism before the outbreak of its local symptom, is demonstrated, like that of the chancre miasma, by the complete disappearance of the discoloration on the spot of the skin, which discoloration remains after every merely local destruction of the fig-wart as a sign of the unextirpated sycosis.

* A master tiler from the Saxon-Erz Mountains, whose dissolute wife had infected him with a venereal disease in his genitals, concerning which it was not apparent from his description whether it was a chancre or a fig-wart, had been so maltreated by violent Mercurial remedies that he had lost his uvula, and his nose was so affected that the fleshy parts had mostly been eaten away, and the remaining part was swollen and inflamed and pierced like a honeycomb with ulcers. This was attended with great pain and an intolerably fetid smell. In addition he had a psoric ulcer on the leg. The anti-psoric remedies improved the ulcers up to a certain degree; they healed the ulcer on the leg, they took away the burning pain and most of the fetid smell of the nose; also the remedies given to cure the sycosis caused some improvement—but as to the sum total nothing further was effected until he received a small dose of Protoxide of Mercury, after which everything was fully healed and he was restored to full health, excepting the irreparable loss of his nose.

PSORA.

I think it necessary before proceeding to the doctrine of the *third* chronic miasma, the most important of all, Psora, to premise the following general remark:

For the infection with the only three known chronic miasmatic diseases there is usually needed but one moment; but the development of this tinder of infection, so that it becomes a general disease of the entire organism, needs a longer time. Not until a certain number of days have elapsed, when the miasmatic disease has received its complete internal development in the whole man—not until then, from the fulness of internal suffering, the local symptom breaks forth, destined by a kind nature to take upon itself in a certain sense the internal disease, and in so far to divert it in a palliative manner and to soothe it, so that it may not be able to injure and endanger the vital economy too much. The local symptom has its place on the least dangerous part of the body, the external skin, and, indeed, on that part of the skin where, during the infection, the miasma had touched the nearest nerves.

This process of nature, which repeats itself continually and evermore in the same manner in chronic miasmata,—aye, even in those which are acute and constant,—ought not to have escaped the penetration of physicians, at least not in venereal diseases, to the treatment of which they have applied themselves now for more than three hundred years; and then they could not have avoided drawing a conclusion as to the process of nature in the other two chronic miasmata. It was, therefore, irrational and unpardonably thoughtless of them to suppose that every chancre evolved by the organism after several days, often after quite a number of days, as the result of the completed internal malady, was a thing merely adventitious from without and situated on the skin without any internal connection, so that it might be simply removed by cauterizing, "so as to prevent the poison from the chancre (*scilicet*) from being absorbed into the internal parts, and thus from causing man to be afflicted with the venereal disease." Irrational and unpardonably thoughtless was this false idea of the origin of the venereal chancre, which caused the injurious practice of the external cauterization of the chancre, producing as its unavoidable, shameful effect, the breaking out of the venereal disease from the internal which has continued in its diseased state. This has been the case in several hundred thousands of cases these last three centuries. Just as irrational and thoughtless is the notion of physicians of the old school, even of the most modern times, that itch is *merely a disease of the skin*, in which the internal portion of the body takes no part. According to this groundless supposition, therefore, nothing better can be done than to remove this ailment from the surface of the skin, although the extirpation of the internal Psora disease which causes the cutaneous eruption is necessary as an aid, and when this is cured also the cutaneous ailment, being the necessary consequence of the internal disease, will naturally disappear—*cessante causa, cessat effectus.*

For in its complete state, *i. e.*, so long as the original eruption is still present on the skin so as to assuage the internal malady, the entire disease of the Psora may be cured most easily, quickly and surely.

But when by the destruction of this original cutaneous eruption, which acts vicariously for the internal malady, it has been robbed then the Psora is put in the unnatural position of dominating in a merely one-sided manner the internal finer parts of the whole organism, and thus of being compelled to develop its secondary symptoms.

How important and necessary the cutaneous eruption is for the original Psora, and how carefully in the only thorough cure of itch, that is, the internal cure, every external removal of the eruption must be avoided, we may see from the fact that the most severe chronic ailments have followed as secondary symptoms of the internal Psora after the original itch-eruption has been driven out, and that when, in consequence of a great revolution in the organism, this itching eruption reappears on the skin, the secondary symptoms are so suddenly removed, that these grievous ailments, often of many years' standing, are wont to disappear, at least temporarily, as if by a miracle. See the before quoted observations of older physicians, Nos. 1, 3, 5, 6, 8, (9), 16, (17), (21), 23, 33, 35, 39, 41, 54, 58, 60, 72, 81, 87, 89, 94.

But let no one suppose that an internal Psora, which, after the external destruction of the original cutaneous eruption, has broken out into secondary chronic ailments, can, through the reappearance of such an itch-like eruption on the skin, come into just as normal a state as before, or that it can be cured just as easily as if it were still the original eruption and as if this had not been as yet removed.

This is not at all the case. Even the eruption following immediately after the infection has no such unchanging constancy and pertinacity on the skin as the chancre and the figwarts show on the spots where they first appear,* but not infrequently disappears from the skin also from other causes† than from artificial remedies used purposely for its destruction, and so also from other causes unknown.‡

So that the physician must not waste any time even in the original eruption, if he would complete the cure while the itch disease is still entire, by the use of internal anti-psoric remedies. Such a respite can be expected still less in this secondary eruption, which has been brought out on the skin by any cause after the local extirpation of the eruption; for the second eruption is wont to be far more inconstant and changeable, so that it often passes away on much slighter provocation in a few days—a proof that it lacks much of the complete quality of the primitive itch-eruption, so that

*Neither of these ever passes away of itself, unless destroyed externally on purpose, or the entire disease is healed internally.

†*E. g.*, through cold, see No. 67 of the above-named observations; through smallpox, No. 39; through warm baths, No. 35.

‡See Nos. 9, 17, 26 (36), 50, 58, 61, 64, 65, in which observations it may be seen at the same time that after such disappearances of the original itch eruption without appreciable cause just as many ill effects are wont to follow as when it has been driven away artificially through local applications.

the physician cannot count on it in the thorough cure of the Psora.

This proneness to change in the itch-like eruption which has been called a second time to the skin, seems evidently to be caused by the fact that the internal Psora, after the destruction of the original itch-eruption, is unable to give to the secondary eruption the full qualities belonging to the primary eruption, and is already much more inclined to unfold itself in a variety of other chronic diseases; wherefore a thorough cure is now much more difficult, and is simply to be conducted as if directed against the internal Psora.

The cure is not, therefore, advanced by producing such a secondary eruption through internal remedies, as has sometimes been effectually attempted (see Nos. 3, 9, 59, 89); or by its re-appearance through other unknown causes (see Nos. 1, 5, 6, 8, 16, 23, 28, 29, 33, 35, 39, 41, 54, 58, 60, 72, 80, 81, 87, 89, 94), or, especially, through the help of a fever (see No. 64, also 55, 56, 74). Such a secondary eruption is always very transitory, and so unreliable and rare that we cannot build our hope of cure on it, nor expect from it the advancement of any thorough cure.

But even if, by any means, such a secondary eruption might, after a fashion, be produced, and even were it in our power to retain it on the skin for a longer period we cannot at all count on it for an assistance in the cure of the whole psoric malady.*

---

*There was a time when, not yet fully convinced of this fact, I thought that the cure of the entire Psora might be rendered easier by an artificial renewal of the cutaneous eruption effected through a sort of checking of the perspiratory function of the skin, so as to

It remains, therefore, an established truth that the cure of the entire destructive Psora through antipsoric remedies is effected most easily only while the original eruption of itch is still present. From this it again appears how unconscionable it is of the allopathic physicians to destroy the primitive itch eruption through

---

excite it homœopathically to the reproduction of the eruption. For this purpose I found most serviceable the wearing of a plaster mostly on the back (but where practicable also on other portions of the skin); the plaster was prepared by *gently* heating six ounces of Burgundy pitch, into which, after removing it from the fire, an ounce of turpentine produced from the larch tree (called Venetian turpentine) was stirred until it was perfectly mixed. A portion of this was spread on a chamois skin (as being the softest) and laid on while still warm. Instead of this there might also be used so-called tree-wax (made of yellow wax and common turpentine), or also taffeta covered with elastic resin; showing that the itching eruption evolved is not due to any irritation caused by the substance applied, nor does the plaster first mentioned cause either eruption or itching on the skin of a person who is not psoric. I discovered that this method is the most effective to cause such an activity of the skin. Yet, despite all the patience of the sick persons (no matter how much they might internally be affected with the Psora), I never could evolve a complete eruption of itch, least of all one that would remain for a time on the skin. What could be effected was only that some itching pustules appeared, which soon vanished again when the plaster was left off. More frequently there ensued a moist soreness of the skin, or at best a more or less violent itching of the skin, which, in rare cases, extended also to the other parts not covered by the plaster. This, indeed, would cause for a time a striking alleviation of even the most severe chronic diseases flowing from a psoric source, *e. g.*, suppuration of the lungs. But this much could not be attained on the skin of many patients (frequently all that could be attained was a moderate or small amount of itching), or, again, if I could produce a violent itching, this frequently became too unbearable for the

local applications instead of completely eradicating this grave disease from the whole living organism by a cure from within, which at that stage is as yet very easy, and by thus choking off in advance all the wretched consequences that we must expect from this malady if uncured, *i. e.*, all the secondary, chronic, nameless sufferings which follow it.

The excuse of the private physician (for the physician at the hospital has no excuse at all) amounts to nothing. He will say, indeed: "If it is not known—and hardly ever does it become demonstrably known—where, when, at what occasion and from what person avowedly suffering from itch the infection has been derived, then he could not discover from the present, and often insignificant little eruption whether it was real itch; so he was not to be blamed for the evil consequences, if he supposed it to be something else and endeavored to remove it from the skin as soon as possible by a lotion of lead solution, or an ointment of cadmia, or white precipitate of mercury, according to the wishes of the aristocratic parents."

---

patient to sustain it for a time sufficient to produce an internal cure. When the plaster then was removed in order to relieve him, even the most violent itching, together with the eruption present, disappeared very soon, and the cure had not been essentially advanced by it; this confirms the observation made above, that the eruption, if evolved a second time (and so also the itching reproduced), had not by any means the full characteristics of the eruption of the itch which had originally been repressed, and was therefore of little assistance in the real advancement of a thorough cure of the Psora through internal remedies, while the little aid afforded loses all value owing to the often unbearable infliction of the artificially produced eruption and itching of the skin and the weakening of the whole body, which is inseparable from the titillating pain.

This excuse, as above said, amounts to nothing. For, *first* of all, *no cutaneous eruption, of whatever kind it may be*, ought to be expelled through external means by any physician who wishes to act conscientiously and rationally.* The human skin does not evolve of itself, without the co-operation of the rest of the living whole, any eruption, nor does it become sick in any way, without being induced and compelled to it by the general diseased state, by the lack of normality in the whole organism. In every case there is at the bottom a disorderly state of the whole internal living organism, which state must first be considered; and therefore the eruption is only to be removed by internal healing and curative remedies which change the state of the whole; then also the eruption which is based on the internal disease will be cured and healed of itself, without the help of any external remedy, and frequently more quickly than it could be done by external remedies.

Secondly, even if the physician should not have presented to him the original, undestroyed form of the eruption,—*i. e.*, the pustule of itch which in the beginning is transparent, then quickly filled with pus, with a narrow red margin all around it,—even if the eruption should consist only of small granules like the miliary eruption, or appear like scattered little pimples or little scabs, still he cannot for a moment be in doubt as to whether the eruption is itch, if the child or even the suckling only a few days old, uninterruptedly rubs and scratches the spot, or if it is an adult,

* See "Organon of the Healing Art," fifth edition, § 187–203.

when he complains of the titillation of a voluptuously itching eruption (or even only a few pimples) which is unbearable without scratching, especially in the evening and at night, and when this is followed by a burning pain. In such a case we can never doubt as to the infection with itch, though in genteel and wealthy families we can seldom secure the information and the certainty as to how, where and from whom the infection has been derived; for there are innumerable imperceptible occasions whereby this infection may be received, as taught above.

Now when the family physician notices this in time, then without any internal application, the simple dose of one or two pills as large as poppy-seeds, moistened with the potentized sulphur in alcohol, as described below, will fully and abundantly suffice to cure a child and to deliver it from the entire disease of itch, both the eruption and the internal itch malady (Psora).

The homœopathic physician in his private practice seldom gets to see and to treat an eruption of itch spread over a considerable part of the skin and coming from a fresh infection. The patients on account of the intolerable itching either apply to some old woman, or to the druggist or the barber, who, one and all, come to their aid with a remedy which, as they suppose, is immediately effective (*e. g.*, lard mixed with flowers of sulphur). Only in the practice of the barracks, of prisons, hospitals, penitentiaries and orphan asylums those infected have to apply to the resident physician, if the surgeon of the house does not anticipate him.

Even in the most ancient times when itch occurred,

for it did not everywhere degenerate into leprosy, it was acknowledged that there was a sort of specific virtue against itch in *sulphur;* but they knew of no other way of applying it, but to destroy the itch through an external application of it, even as is done now by the greater part of the modern physicians of the old school. A. C. Celsus has several ointments and salves (V. 28), some of which consist merely of sulphur mixed with tar, while others contain also compounds of copper and other substances; these he prescribes for the expulsion of itch, and this he supposes to be its cure. So also the most ancient physicians, like the moderns, prescribed for their itch patients baths of warm sulphurous mineral water. Such patients are usually also delivered from their eruption by these external sulphur remedies. But that their patients were not really cured thereby, became manifest, even to them, from the more severe ailments that followed, such as general dropsy, with which an Athenian was afflicted when he drove out his severe eruption of itch by bathing in the warm sulphur baths of the island of Melos (now called Milo), and of which he died. This is recorded by the author of Book V., Epidemion, which has been received among the writings of Hippocrates (some three hundred years before Celsus).

Internally the ancient physicians gave no Sulphur in itch, because they, like the moderns, did not see that this miasmatic disease was, at the same time *and specially*, an internal disease.

Modern physicians have never given Sulphur *only*, and internally, to cure the itch, because they have never recognized the itch disease as being also an internal *and*, indeed, *chiefly* internal disease. They only gave it in connection with the external means of driving away the itch, and, indeed, in doses which would act as purgatives,—ten, twenty and thirty grains at a dose, frequently repeated,—so that it never became manifest how useful or how injurious this internal application of such large doses, in connection with the external application, had been; *at least* the whole itch disease (Psora) *could never* be thoroughly healed thereby. The external driving out of the eruption was simply advanced by it as by any other purgative, and with the same injurious effects as if no Sulphur at all had been used internally. For even if Sulphur is used only internally, but in the above described large doses, without any external destructive means, it can never thoroughly heal Psora; partly because in order to cure as an antipsoric and homœopathic medicine, it must be given only in the smallest doses of a potentized preparation, while in larger and more frequent doses the crude Sulphur* in some cases increases the malady

* Here it is proper to subjoin the words of an impartial and even practical connoisseur of Homœopathy, the deep-thinking, many-sided scholar and indefatigable investigator of truth, Count Buquoy, in his *Anregungen für ph. w. Forschungen* (Leipzig, 1825, p. 386 sgg.). After assuming that a drug, which in a normal state of health causes the symptoms *a*, *b*, *g*,—in analogy with other physiological phenomena, produces the symptoms *x*, *y*, *z*, which appear in an abnormal state of health—can act upon this abnormal state in such a way that the disease symptoms *x*, *y*, *z*, are transformed into the drug symptoms *a*, *b*, *g*, which latter have the peculiar characteristic of temporariness or transitoriness; he then continues: "This transitory character belongs to the group of

or at least adds a new malady; partly because the vital force expels it as a violently aggressive remedy through purging stools or by means of vomiting, without having put its healing power to any use.

Now if, as experience teaches, not even the fresh itch disease which is the most easy to cure of all, *i. e.*, the internal, recently formed Psora together with the external, recent eruption, can be thoroughly healed by external applications accompanied by large quantities of flowers of Sulphur, it may easily be seen, that the Psora, after it has been deprived of its eruption and has become merely internal and inveterate, having developed secondary ailments and thus having changed into chronic diseases of various kinds, for the same reason can be just as little cured by a quantity of Sulphur flowers, or by a number of baths in sulphurous mineral waters, or on the other hand, by simultaneously drinking the same or a similar water; in a word, it cannot be cured by a superabundance and frequent repetition of this remedy, although it is of itself anti-psoric.* It is true that many such chronic

---

symptoms of the medicine *a, b, g*, which is substituted for the group of symptoms belonging to the disease, merely because the medicine is used in an *extraordinarily small* dose. Should the homœopathic physician give the patient *too large* a dose of the homœopathic remedy indicated, the disease *x, y, z*, may, indeed, be transformed into the other, *i. e.*, into *a, b, g*, but the new disease *now sits just as firmly fixed* as the former *x, y, z;* so that the organism *can just as little free itself from the disease a, b, g*, as it was able to throw off the original disease *x, y, z*. If a *very large* dose is given, then *a new*, often *very dangerous disease* is produced, or the organism does its utmost to free itself very quickly from the poison (through diarrhœa, vomiting, etc.)."

* Used in small doses, Sulphur as one of the anti-psoric remedies

patients by the first treatment at the baths seem to get rid for some time of the symptoms of their disease (therefore we see an incredible throng of many thousands, suffering from innumerable different chronic ailments at Teplitz, Baden, Aix-la-Chapelle, Neundorf, Warmbrunn, etc.); yet they are not on that account restored to health, but instead of the original chronic (psoric) disease, they have for a time come under the dominion of a Sulphur disease (another, perhaps more bearable, malady). This in time passes away, when the Psora again lifts its head, either with the same morbid symptoms as before, or with others similar but gradually more troublesome than the first, or with symptoms developing in nobler parts of the organism. Ignorant persons will rejoice in the latter case, that their former disease at least has passed away, and they hope that the new disease also may be removed by another journey to the same baths. They do not know, that their changed morbid state is merely a transformation of the same Psora; but they always find out by experience, that their second tour to the baths causes even less alleviation, or, indeed, if the Sulphur baths are used in still greater number, that the second trial causes aggravation.

Thus we see that either the excessive use of Sul-

---

will not fail to make a brief beginning of a cure of the chronic (non-venereal and therefore psoric) diseases. I know a physician in Saxony who gained a great reputation by merely adding to his prescription in nearly all chronic diseases flowers of Sulphur, and this without knowing a reason for it. This *in the beginning* of such treatments is wont to produce a strikingly beneficent effect, but of course *only* in the beginning, and therefore after that his help was at an end.

phur in all its forms, or the frequent repetition of its use by allopathic physicians in the treatment of a multitude of chronic diseases (the secondary psoric ailments) have taken away from it all value and use; and we may well assert that, to this day, hardly anything but injury has been done by allopathic physicians through the use of Sulphur.

But even supposing that anyone should desire to make the only correct use of Sulphur in this kind of disease, it will seldom be possible to do this with the same desired success as where the homœopathic physician finds a recent case of the itch-disease with its still existing eruption. Even when, owing to its undeniable antipsoric effects, Sulphur may be able of itself to make the beginning of a cure, after the external expulsion of the eruption, either with the still hidden and latent Psora or when this has more or less developed and broken out into its varied chronic diseases, it can nevertheless be but rarely made use of for this purpose, because its powers have usually been already exhausted because it has been given to the patient already before by allopathic physicians for one purpose or another, perhaps has been already given repeatedly; but Sulphur, like most of the antipsoric remedies in the treatment of a developed Psora that has become chronic, can hardly be used three or four times (even after the intervening use of other antipsoric remedies) without causing the cure to retrograde.

The cure of an old Psora that has been deprived of its eruption, whether it may be latent and quiescent or already broken out into chronic diseases, can never be accomplished with Sulphur alone, nor with sulphur-baths, either natural or artificial.

Here I may mention the curious circumstance that in general—with the exception of the recent itch-disease still attended with its unrepressed cutaneous eruption, and which is so easily cured from within*—every other psoric diathesis, *i. e.*, the Psora that is still latent within, as well as the Psora that has developed into one of the innumerable chronic diseases springing from it, is very seldom cured by any single antipsoric remedy, but requires the use of several of these remedies—in the worst cases the use of quite a number of them—one after the other, for its perfect cure.

This circumstance need not astonish us when we consider that the Psora is a chronic miasma of quite peculiar and especial character, which in several thousands of years has passed through several millions of human organisms, and must have assumed such a vast extension of varied symptoms—the elements of those innumerable, chronic, non-venereal ailments, under which mankind now groans—and could transmute itself into such an indefinite multitude of forms differing from one another as it gradually ultimated itself in the various bodily constitutions of individual men who differed from one another in their domiciles, their climatic peculiarities, their education, habits, occupations.

*Recent itch-disease with its still present cutaneous eruption has been cured at times without any external remedy by even *one* very small dose of a properly potentized preparation of Sulphur, and thus within two, three or four weeks; once a dose of one-half grain of Carbo vegetabilis, potentized a million fold, sufficed for a family of seven persons, and three times a like dose of as highly potentized Sepia was sufficient.

†*I. e.*, occupations which called more fully into play one or another organ of the body, one or another function of the spirit and mind.

modes of life and of diet, and was moulded by varying bodily and psychic relations. It is, therefore, not strange that one single and only medicine is insufficient to heal the entire Psora and all its forms, and that it requires several medicines in order to respond, by the artificial morbid effects peculiar to each, to the unnumbered host of Psora symptoms, and thus to those of all chronic (non-venereal) diseases and to the entire Psora, and to do this in a curative homœopathic manner.*

It is only, therefore, as already mentioned, when the eruption of itch is still in its prime and the infection is in consequence still recent, that the complete cure can be effected by Sulphur alone, and then at times with but a single dose. I leave it undecided whether this can be done in every case of itch still in full eruption on the skin, because the ages of the eruption of itch-infecting patients is quite various. For if the eruption has been on the skin for some time (although it may not have been treated with external repressive remedies), it will of itself begin to recede gradually from the skin. Then the internal Psora has already in part gained the upper hand; the cutaneous eruption is then no more so completely vicarious, and ailments of another kind appear, partly as the signs of a latent Psora, partly as chronic diseases developed from the internal Psora. In such a case Sulphur alone (as little as any

*I refrain from hinting through what exertions and through how many careful observations, investigations, reflections and varied experiments I have finally succeeded after eleven years in filling up the great chasm in the edifice of the homœopathic healing art, the cure of the innumerable chronic diseases, and thus in completing as far as possible the blessings which this art has in store for suffering humanity.

other single antipsoric remedy) is usually no longer sufficient to produce a complete cure, and the other antipsoric remedies, one or another, according to the remaining symptoms, must be called upon to give their homœopathic aid.

The homœopathic medical treatment of the countless chronic diseases (non-venereal and, therefore, of psoric origin) agrees essentially in its general features with the homœopathic treatment of human diseases as taught in the *Organon of the Art of Healing*. I shall now indicate what is especially to be considered in the treatment of chronic diseases.

As to the *diet and mode of living* of patients of this kind I shall only make some general remarks, leaving the special application in any particular case to the judgment of the homœopathic practitioner. Of course everything that would hinder the cure must also in these cases be removed. But since we have here to treat lingering, sometimes very tedious, diseases, which cannot be quickly removed, and since we often have cases of patients in middle life and also in old age, in various relations of life, which can seldom be totally changed, either in the case of rich people or in the case of persons of small means, or even with the poor, therefore limitations and modifications of the strict mode of life as regularly prescribed by Homœopathy must be allowed in order to make possible the cure of such tedious diseases with individuals so very different. A strict, homœopathic diet and mode of living does not *cure* chronic patients, as our opponents pretend in order to diminish the merits of Homœopathy, but the main cause is the medical treatment. This may be seen in the case of the many patients who, trusting these false allegations, have for years observed the most strict homœopathic diet without being able thereby to diminish appreciably their chronic disease; this rather increasing in spite of the diet, as all diseases of a chronic miasmatic nature do from their nature.

Owing to these causes, therefore, and in order to make the cure possible, the homœopathic practitioner must yield to circumstances in his prescriptions as to *diet* and *mode of living*, and in so doing he will much more surely, and therefore more completely, reach the aim of healing than by an obstinate insistence on strict rules, which in many cases cannot be obeyed.

The daily laborer, if his strength allows, should continue his labor; the artisan, his handiwork; the farmer, so far as he is able, his field work; the mother of the family, her domestic occupations according to her strength; only labors that would interfere with the health of healthy persons should be interdicted. This must be left to the intelligence of the rational physician.

The class of men who are usually occupied, not with bodily labor, but with fine work in their rooms, usually with sedentary work, should be directed during their cure to walk more in the open air, without, on that account, setting their work altogether aside.

Persons belonging to the higher classes should also be urged to take walks more than is their custom. The physician may allow this class the innocent amusement of moderate and becoming dancing, amusements in the country that are reconcilable with a strict diet, also social meetings with acquaintances, where conversation is the chief amusement; he will not keep them from enjoying harmless music or from listening to lectures which are not too fatiguing; he can permit the theatre only exceptionally, but he can never allow the playing of cards. The physician will moderate too frequent riding and driving, and should know how to banish intercourse which should prove to be morally and psychically injurious, as this is also physically injurious. The flirtations and empty excitations of sensuality between the sexes, the reading of indelicate novels and poems of a like character, as well as superstitious and enthusiastic books, are to be altogether interdicted.*

Scholars ought also to be induced to (moderately) exercise in the open air, and in bad weather to do some light mechanical work in doors; but during the medical treatment mental occupation should be limited to work from memory, since straining the head by reading is hardly ever to be allowed, or at least only with great limitation and a strict definition as to the quantity and quality of what is read, *i. e.*, in treating any

* Physicians frequently wish to assume importance by forbidding without exception all sexual intercourse to chronic patients who are married. But if both parties are able and disposed to it, such an interdict is, to say the least, ridiculous, as it neither can nor will be obeyed (without causing a greater misfortune in the family). No legislature should give laws that cannot be kept nor controlled, or which would cause even greater mischief if kept. If one party is incapable of sexual intercourse, this of itself will stop such intercourse. But of all functions in marriage such intercourse is what may least be commanded or forbidden. Homœopathy only interferes in this matter through medicines, so as to make the party that is incapable of sexual intercourse capable of it, through antipsoric (or anti-syphilitic) remedies, or, on the other hand, to reduce an excitable consort's morbidity to its natural tone.

of the more severe chronic diseases. In mental disorders it can never be allowed.

All classes of chronic patients must be forbidden the use of any domestic remedies or the use of any medicines on their own account. With the higher classes, perfumeries, scented waters, tooth-powders and other medicines for the teeth must also be forbidden. If the patient has been accustomed for a long time to woolen under-clothing, the homœopathic physician cannot suddenly make a change, but as the disease diminishes the woolen under-garments may in warm weather be first changed to cotton, and then, in warm weather, the patient can pass to linen. Fontanels can be stopped, in chronic diseases of any moment, only when the internal cure has already made progress, especially with patients of advanced age.

The physician cannot yield to the request of patients for the continuance of their customary home-baths, but a quick ablution, as much as cleanliness may demand from time to time, may be allowed; nor can he permit any venesection or cupping, however much the patient may declare that he has become accustomed thereto.

As to *diet*, all classes of men who wish to be cured of a lingering disease, can suffer some limitation, if the chronic disease does not consist of an ailment of the abdomen; with the lower classes there need be no very strict limitations, especially if the patient is able to remain at work in his trade, thus giving motion to the body. The poor man can recover health even with a diet of salt and bread, and neither the moderate use of potatoes, flour-porridge nor fresh cheese will hinder his recovery; only let him limit the condiments of onions and pepper with his meagre diet.

He who cares for his recovery can find dishes, even at the king's table, which answer all the requirements of a natural diet.

Most difficult for a homœopathic physician is the decision as to drinks. Coffee has in great part the injurious effects on the health of body and soul which I have described in my little book (*Wirkungen des Kaffees* [Effects of Coffee], Leipzig, 1803); but it has become so much of a habit and a necessity to the greater part of the so-called enlightened nations that it will be as difficult to extirpate as prejudice and superstition, unless the homœopathic physician in the cure of chronic diseases insist on a general, absolute interdict. Only young people up to the twentieth year, or at most up to the thirtieth, can be suddenly deprived of it without any particular disadvantage; but with persons over thirty and forty years, if they have used coffee from their childhood, it is better to propose to discontinue it gradually and every day to drink somewhat less; when lo and behold! most of them leave it off at once, and they will do so without any peculiar trouble (except, perhaps, for a few days at the commencement). As late as six years ago I still supposed that older persons who are unwilling to do without it, might be allowed to use it in a small quantity. But I have since then become convinced that even a long-continued habit cannot make it harmless, and as the physician can only permit what is best for his patient, it must remain as an established rule that chronic patients must altogether give up this part of their diet, which is insidiously injurious; and this the patients, high or low, who have the proper confidence in their physician, when it is properly represented to them, almost without exception, do willingly and gladly, to the great improvement of their health. Rye or wheat, roasted like coffee in a drum and then boiled and prepared like coffee, has both in smell and taste much resemblance to coffee; and rich and poor are using this substitute willingly in several countries.

The like may be said concerning the expensive and so-called fine sorts, as well as concerning the cheap sorts of Chinese tea which so flatteringly allures the nerves and so secretly and inevitably infests and weakens them. Even when made very weak and when only a little is drank only once a day it is never harmless, neither with younger persons nor with older ones who have used it since their childhood; and they must instead of it use some harmless warm drink. Patients, according to my extensive experience, are also willing to follow the advice of their faithful adviser, the physician in whom they have confidence, when this advice is fortified with reason.

With respect to the limitation in wine the practitioner can be far more lenient, since with chronic patients it will be hardly ever necessary to altogether forbid it. Patients who from their youth up have been accustomed to a plentiful use of pure* wine cannot give it up at once entirely, and this the less the older they are. To do so would produce a sudden

---

*Even for men in quite good health it is improper and in many ways injurious to drink pure wine as a customary beverage, and morality only permits its use in small quantities at festive occasions. A youth cannot keep his sexual desires under control up to his marriage unless he altogether avoids banquets. Gonorrhœa and chancre are due to such excesses.

sinking of their strength and an obstruction to their cure, and might even endanger their life. But they will be satisfied to drink it during the first weeks mixed with equal parts of water, and later, gradually wine mixed with two, three and four and finally with five and six parts of water and a little sugar. The latter mixtures may be allowed all chronic patients as their usual beverage.

More absolutely necessary in the cure of the chronic diseases is the giving up of whisky or brandy. This will require, however, as much consideration in diminishing the quantity used, as firmness in executing it. Where the strength appreciably diminishes at giving it up totally, a small portion of good, pure wine must be used instead of it for a little while, but later, wine mixed with several parts of water, according to circumstances.

Since, according to an inviolable law of nature, our vital force always produces in the human organism the opposite of the impressions caused by physical and medicinal potencies in all the cases in which there are such opposites, it may easily be understood, as accurate observation also testifies, that spirituous liquors, after having simulated refreshment and heightened vital warmth immediately after partaking them, must have just the opposite after-effects, owing to this opposite reaction of the vital force of the organism. Weakness and a diminution of the vital warmth are the inevitable consequences of their use—states which ought to be removed as far as possible from the chronic patient by every true physician. Only an allopath who has never accustomed himself to observation and to reflection, and who is unwilling to acknowledge the injurious effects of his palliatives, can advise his chronic patients to daily drink strong, pure wine to strengthen themselves; a genuine Homœopath will never do this (*sed ex ungue leonem!*).

The permission of beer is quite questionable! Since the artifices of brewers in modern times seem to intend, by their addition of vegetable substances to the extract of malt, not only to prevent it from souring, but also and especially to tickle the palate and to cause intoxication, without any regard to the injurious qualities of these malignant additions which often deeply undermine the health when daily used, and which cannot be discovered by any inspection, the honest physician cannot allow his patient to drink whatsoever is called *beer;* for even the white beer (thin beer) and the porter, which on account of their lack of bitterness seem so harmless, not infrequently have narcotic ingredients added to give them the much-liked intoxicating quality in spite of their diminished quantity of malt.

Among the articles of diet which are generally injurious to chronic patients are also all dishes containing vinegar or citric acid. These are especially apt to cause disagreeable sensations and troubles in those afflicted with nervous and abdominal ailments. They also either antagonize or excessively increase the effects of several medicines. For such patients also very acid fruit (as sour cherries, unripe gooseberries and currants) are to be allowed only in very small quantities, and sweet fruits only in moderate quantity; so also baked prunes as a palliative are not to be advised to those inclined to constipation. To the latter, as also to those suffering from weak digestion, veal which is too young is not serviceable. Those whose sexual powers are low should limit themselves in eating young chickens and eggs, and should avoid the irritating spice of vanilla, also truffles and caviare, which as palliatives hinder a cure. Ladies with scanty menses must avoid the use of saffron and cinnamon for the same reason; persons with weak stomachs should avoid cinnamon, cloves, amomum, pepper, ginger and bitter substances, which, being palliatives, are also injurious while under homœopathic treatment. Vegetables causing flatulency should be forbidden in all abdominal troubles and where there is an inclination to constipation and costiveness. Beef and good wheat-bread or rye-bread, together with cow's milk and a moderate use of fresh butter, seem to be the most natural and harmless food for men, and also for chronic patients; only little salt should be used. Next to beef in wholesomeness are mutton, venison, grown chickens and young pigeons. The flesh and fat of geese and ducks are even less to be permitted to chronic patients than pork. Pickled and smoked meats should be rarely used and only in small quantities.

Sprinkling chopped raw herbs on soups, putting pot-herbs into vegetables, and eating old, rancid cheese must be avoided.

In using the better quality of fish their preparation should be especially looked to; they had best be prepared by boiling and used sparingly with sauces not much spiced; but no fish dried in the air or smoked;

salt fish (herrings and sardines) only rarely and sparingly.

Moderation in all things, even in harmless ones, is the chief duty of chronic patients.

In considering diet, the use of tobacco should also be carefully considered. Smoking in some cases of chronic disease may be permitted, when the patient has been accustomed to an uninterrupted use of it, and if he does not expectorate; but smoking should always be limited, and more so if the mental activity, sleep, digestion or the evacuations are defective. If evacuations regularly only take place after smoking the use of this palliative must be all the more circumscribed, and the same result must be obtained in a lasting manner through the appropriate antipsoric remedies. More objectionable yet, however, is the using of snuff, which is wont to be abused as a palliative against rheum and obstruction of the nose and insidious inflammation of the eyes, and which being a palliative, is a great hinderance in the cure of chronic diseases; it can, therefore, not be allowed with such patients, but must be diminished every day and at last stopped. An especial reason for this is also that in snuff the medicinal liquors (sauces) with which almost all snuff is medicated touches with its substance the nerves of the inner nose and injures just as if a foreign medicine were taken, which is less the case with the burning, smoking tobacco in which the strength is disintegrated by the heat.

I now pass to the other hinderances to the cure of chronic diseases which must be avoided as far as possible.

All those events in human life which can bring the Psora latent and slumbering within, which has hitherto manifested itself only by some of the signs mentioned above, wherein the patient varies from a state of health, so as to break out into open chronic diseases, these same events if they occur to a person already a chronic patient may not only augment his disease and increase the difficulty of curing it, but if they break in on him violently, may make his disease incurable, if the untoward circumstances are not suddenly changed for the better.

Such events are, however, of very various nature, and therefore of different degrees of injurious influence.

Excessive hardships, laboring in swamps, great bodily injuries and wounds, excess of cold or heat, and even the unsatisfied hunger of poverty and its unwholesome foods, etc., are not by any means very powerful in causing the fearful malady of Psora which lies in ambush, lurking in secret to break forth into serious chronic diseases, nor of great consequence in aggravating a chronic disease already present; yea, an innocent man can, with less injury to his life, pass ten years in bodily torments in the bastile or on the galleys rather than pass some months in all bodily comfort in an unhappy marriage or with a remorseful conscience. A Psora slumbering within, which still allows the favorite of a prince to live with the appearance of almost blooming health, unfolds quickly into a chronic ailment of the body, or distracts his mental organs into insanity, when by a change of fortune he is hurled from his brilliant pinnacle and is exposed to contempt and poverty. The sudden death of a son causes the tender mother, already in ill health, an incurable suppuration of the lungs or a cancer of the breast. A young, affectionate maiden, already hysterical, is thrown into melancholy by a disappointment in love.

How difficult it is, and how seldom will the best anti-psoric treatment do anything to relieve such unfortunates!

By far the most frequent excitement of the slumbering Psora into chronic disease, and the most frequent aggravation of chronic ailments already existing, are caused by grief and vexation.

Uninterrupted grief and vexation very soon increase even the smallest traces of a slumbering Psora into more severe symptoms, and they then develop these into an outbreak of all imaginable chronic sufferings more certainly and more frequently than all other injurious influences operating on the human organism in an average human life; while these two agencies just as surely and frequently augment ailments already existing.

As the good physician will be pleased when he can enliven and keep from ennui the mind of a patient, in order to advance a cure which is not encumbered with such obstructions, he will in such a case feel more than ever the duty incumbent upon him to do all within the power of his influence on the patient and on his relatives and surroundings, in order to relieve him of grief and vexation. This will and must be a chief end of his care and neighborly love.

But if the relations of the patient cannot be improved in this respect, and if he has not sufficient philosophy, religion and power over himself to bear patiently and with equanimity all the sufferings and afflictions for which he is not to blame, and which it is not in his power to change; if grief and vexation continually beat in upon him, and it is out of the power of the physician to effect a lasting removal of these most active destroyers of life, he had better give up the treatment* and leave the patient to his fate, for even the most masterly management of the case with the remedies that are the most exquisite and the best adapted to the bodily ailment will avail nothing, nothing at all, with a chronic patient thus exposed to continual sorrow and vexation, and in whom the vital economy is being destroyed by continuous assaults on the mind. The continuation of the fairest edifice is foolish, when the foundation is being daily undermined, even if but gradually, by the play of the waves.

Almost as near, and often nearer yet, to incurability are the chronic diseases, especially with great and rich men, who for some years, besides the use of mineral baths,† have passed through the hands of various, often

---

*Unless the patient should have little or no cause for his grief and sorrow, or hardly any incitement from without to vexation, and in consequence would need more particularly to be treated with respect to his mental disorder, by means of the anti-psoric remedies, which are at the same time suited to the rest of his chronic disease. Such cases are not only curable, but often even easily curable.

† Every time the baths are used, even when the water is not in itself unsuitable to the ailment, they are to be considered as the use of large doses often repeated of one and the same violently acting medicine, the violent operation of which can seldom be salutary, and must often result in the aggravation of the morbid state, yea, even to the patient's utter destruction.

of *many*, allopathic physicians, who have tried on them one after another all the fashionable modes of cure, the remedies which are so boastingly lauded in England, France and Italy,—all strongly acting mixtures. By so many unsuitable medicines, which are injurious by their violence and their frequent repetition in large doses, the Psora which always lies within, even if not combined with syphilis, becomes every year more incurable, as do also the chronic ailments springing from it; and after the continuation of such irrational medical assaults on the organism for several years it becomes almost quite incurable. It cannot well be decided, since these things take place in the dark, whether these heroic unhomœopathic doses have added, as may be suspected, new ailments to the original disease, which ailments through the largeness of the doses and their frequent repetition have now become lasting and as it were chronic, or whether through abuse there has resulted a crippling of the different faculties of the organism, *i. e.*, those of irritability, of sensation and of reproduction, and so (probably from both causes) there has arisen the monster of various ailments, fused into one another, which can no longer be rationally viewed as a simple natural ailment. In short, this many sided disharmony and perversion of parts and of forces most indispensable to life present a chaos of ailments which the homœopathic physician should not lightly declare curable.

By such treatments, which are incapable of curing the original disease, but are exhausting and debilitating, the aggravation of the Psora is not only hastened from within, but new artificial and threatening ailments are generated by such delusive allopathic cures, so that the vital force, thus attacked from two sides, often is unable to escape.

If in such cases the sad consequences of these indirect assaults of the old methods of cure were dynamic disturbances only, they would surely either disappear of themselves when the treatment is discontinued, or they ought at least to be extinguished again effectively through homœopathic medicines. But this is not at all the case; they do not yield. Very likely by these indirect, continuous and repeated assaults on the sensitive, irritable fiber by such injudicious medicinal disease-potencies, which are given in large doses frequently repeated, the vital force is obliged to meet this attack and to endeavor either to dynamically change these tender internal organs which are assaulted so mercilessly, or to reconstruct them materially so as to make them unassailable to such violent attacks, and thus to protect and shield the organism from general destruction. Thus, *e. g.*, this force, which instinctively preserves life, beneficially shields the fine sensitive skin of the hand with a callous covering of hard, horny skin in persons with whom the skin is exposed to frequent injuries during hard labor whereby the skin is injured by hard, scratching materials or by corroding substances. So also in a long continued allopathic treatment, which has no true healing power with respect to the disease, no direct pathic (homœopathic) relation to the parts and processes concerned in the chronic disease, but internally assaults other delicate parts and organs of the body, in such cases the vital force, in order to protect the whole from destruction, dynamically and organically transmutes these fine organs; *i. e.*, either makes them inactive or paralyzes them, or dulls their sensitiveness, or makes them altogether callous. On the one side the most tender fiber is abnormally thickened or hardened, and the more vigorous fibers consumed or annihilated—thus there arise artificially, adventitious organisms, malformations and degenerations, which at post-mortem examinations are cunningly ascribed to the malignancy of the original disease. Such an internal state is not infrequent, and is in many cases incurable. Only where there are still sufficient vital powers in a body not too much bowed down by age (but where under an allopathic régime do we not find the powers wasted?) under favorable external circumstances, the vital force dynamically freed from its original disease by the careful homœopathic (antipsoric) treatment of a practiced physician, may succeed in gradually reasserting itself, and in gradually absorbing and transforming those (often numerous) adventitious secondary formations which it was compelled to form. Such a transformation is, however, only possible to a still energetic vital force, which has been in great part set free from its Psora. Only, however, under favorable external circumstances, and after the lapse of a considerable time and usually in only an imperfect manner, does the vital force succeed in this almost creative endeavor. Experience proves daily that the more zealously the allopath puts into practice in chronic diseases his perverse destructive art (often with great care, industry and persistence), the more he ruins his patients in health and life.

How can perversions, introduced into patients in this manner frequently for years, be transformed in a short time into health even by the best, *i. e.*, the true method of cure, which has never assumed to itself the power of *directly* influencing organic defects?

The physician has to meet in such cases no natural, simple Psoric disease. He can therefore promise an improvement only after a long period of time, but never a full restoration, even if the vital powers are not (as is so frequently the case) altogether wasted; for where this is the case, he would feel compelled to desist from treatment even at the first glance. First the many chronic medicinal diseases which pass over the fluctuating state of health must gradually be removed (perhaps during a several months' stay in the country almost without medicine); or they must depart as of themselves through the activity of the vital force, when the anti-psoric treatment has to some degree begun, with an improved manner of living and a regulated diet. For who could find remedies for all these ailments artificially produced by a confused mass of strong unsuitable medicines? The vital force must first absorb and reform what it has compulsorily deformed, before the true healer will in time see again before him a partially cleared malady similar to the original one, and which he will then be able to combat.*

* On the other hand, the most dreadful diseases of every kind which have not been spoiled by any medical fatuity, in the families of farm laborers and other day laborers, on whom of course no ordinary physician presses his services, are *quite commonly*, almost as if by a miracle, cured by the anti-psoric remedies in a short time, and are transformed into lasting good health.

Woe to the young homœopathic physician who has to found his fame upon the cure of those diseases, of rich and prominent persons, which by a mass of allopathic evil arts have degenerated into such monstrosities! With all his care he will end in failure!

A similar great hindrance to a cure of far-advanced chronic diseases is often found in the debility and weakness into which youths fall who are spoiled by rich parents, being carried away by their superabundance and wantonness, and seduced by wicked companions through destructive passions and excesses, through revelings, abuse of the sexual instinct, gambling, etc. Without the least regard for life and for conscience, bodies orginally robust are debilitated by such vices into mere semblances of humanity, and are besides ruined by perverse treatment of their venereal diseases, so that the Psora, which frequently lurks within, grows up into the most pitiable chronic diseases, which, even if the morality of the patient should have improved, on account of the depressing remorse, and the little remnant of their wasted vital powers, accept antipsoric relief only with the greatest difficulty. Such cases should be undertaken by homœopathic physicians as curable only with the greatest caution and reserve.

But where the above-mentioned often almost insurmountable obstacles to the cure of these innumerable chronic diseases are not present,* there is nevertheless

*One additional obstacle to the homœopathic cure of chronic diseases, and one which is not very rare, but is still usually disregarded, is: *The suppressed sexual instinct* with marriageable persons of either sex, either from non-marriage owing to various causes not

found at times, especially with the lower classes of patients, a peculiar obstruction to the cure, which lies in the source of the malady itself, where the Psora, after repeated infections and a repeated external repression of the resulting eruption, had developed gradually from its internal state into one or more severe chronic ailments. A cure will, indeed, also be certainly effected here, if the above-mentioned obstacles do not prevent, by a judicious use of the antipsoric remedies, but only with much patience and considerable time, and only with patients who observe the directions and who are not too aged or too much debilitated.

But in these difficult cases also the wise arrangement of nature is manifested in aid of our efforts if we only make a good use of the favorable moment offering. For experience informs us that in a case of itch arising from a new infection, even when, after several preceding infections and repressions of the eruption, the Psora has made considerable progress in the production of chronic diseases of many kinds, the itch which has last arisen, if it has only still kept its full primitive eruption unhindered on the skin, may be cured almost as easily as if it were the first and the

---

removable by a physician, or where in married persons sexual intercourse of an infirm wife with a vigorous husband, or of the infirm husband with a vigorous wife has been absolutely and forever interdicted by an injudicious physician, as is not infrequently the case. In such cases a more intelligent physician, recognizing the circumstances and the natural impulse implanted by the Creator, will give his permission and thus most infrequently render curable a multitude of hysterical and hypochondriac states, yea, often even melancholy and insanity.

only one, *i. e.*, usually by merely one or a few doses of the appropriate antipsoric medicine, and that by such a cure the whole Psora of all the preceding infections, together with its outbreaks into chronic ailments, is cured.*

Nevertheless it is not advisable to intentionally cause a new artificial infection with itch, even if the patient felt no repugnance to it (as is, nevertheless, frequently the case) merely on account of the easier cure in that case of the old Psora which had been several times renewed; because in severe chronic diseases of a non-venereal and therefore psoric origin,—as *e. g.*, suppuration of the lungs, a complete paralyzation of one or another part of the body, etc.,—the itch miasma rarely retains its hold, and, as far as experience shows, it clings less when caused by an artificial inoculation than when it originates from an accidental, unintentional infection.

I have little further to say to the physician already skilled in the homœopathic art as to how he is to operate in the cure of chronic diseases, except to direct im to the antipsoric remedies appended to this work;

* The same is the case, according to the merciful arrangement of nature, with syphilis, where, after a local destruction of the chancre or the bubo and after a consequent breaking out of the venereal disease, a new infection takes place. The new infection, while the chancre remains undisturbed, may be cured, together with the venereal disease sprung from the former infection, just as easily by a single dose of the best mercurial preparation, as if the first chancre were still present,—provided that no complication with either of the other two chronic miasmata, especially the psoric, has taken place; for in such a case, as has been mentioned above, the Psora must first be removed.

for he will know how to use these remedies for this noble end successfully. I have only to add a few *cautions.*

First of all, the great truth is established that all chronic ailments, all great, and the greatest, long continuing diseases (excepting the few venereal ones) spring from Psora alone and only find their thorough cure in the cure of the Psora; they are, consequently, to be healed mostly only by antipsoric remedies, *i. e.*, by those remedies which in their provings as to their pure action on the healthy human body manifest most of the symptoms which are most frequently perceived in latent as well as in developed Psora.

The homœopathic physician, therefore, in curing a chronic (non-venereal) disease, and in all and in every symptom, ailment and disorder arising in this disease, no matter what seductive name these may have in common life or in pathology, will usually and especially look to the use of an antipsoric medicine selected according to strictly homœopathic rules, in order to surely attain his end.

Let him not think, while a well-chosen antipsoric medicine is acting and the patient some day feels a moderate headache, or else a moderate ailment, that he must give the patient at once some other medicine, whether an antipsoric or another remedy; or if perchance a sore throat should arise, that he must give another remedy, or on account of diarrhœa, or another on account of some moderate pain in one part or another, etc.

No! the homœopathic antipsoric medicine having been chosen as well as possible to suit the morbid symptoms, and given in the appropriate potency and in the proper dose, the physician should *as a rule* allow it to finish its action without disturbing it by an intervening remedy.

For if the symptoms occurring during the action of the remedy have also occurred, if not in the last few weeks, at least now and then some weeks before, or some months before in a similar manner, then such occurrences are merely a homœopathic excitation, through the medicine, of some symptom not quite unusual to this disease, of something which had perhaps been more frequently troublesome before, and they are a sign that this medicine acts deeply into the very essence of this disease, and that consequently it will be more effective in the future. The medicine, therefore, should be allowed to continue and exhaust its action undisturbed, without giving the least medicinal substance between its doses.

But if the symptoms are different and had never before occurred, or never in this way, therefore, are peculiar to this medicine and not to be expected in the process of the disease, but trifling, the action of the medicine ought not for the present to be interrupted. Such symptoms frequently pass off without interrupting the helpful activity of the remedy; but if they are of a burdensome intensity, they are not to be endured; in such a case they are a sign that the antipsoric medicine was not selected in the correct homœopathic manner. Its action must then be checked by an antidote, or when the antidote to it is known, another antipsoric medicine more accurately answering its symptoms must be given in its place; in this case these false symptoms may continue a few more days, or they may return, but they will soon come to a final end and be replaced by a better help.

Least of all, need we to be concerned when the usual customary symptoms are aggravated and show most prominently on the first days, and again on some of the following days, but gradually less and less. This so-called homœopathic aggravation is a sign of an incipient cure (of the symptoms thus aggravated at present), which may be expected with certainty.

But if these aggravated original symptoms appear on subsequent days still of the same strength as at the beginning, or even with an increased severity, it is a sign that the dose of this antipsoric remedy, although properly selected according to homœopathic principles, was too large, and it is to be apprehended that no cure will be affected by it; because the medicine in so large a dose is able to establish a disease, which in some respects, indeed, is similar to it; with respect to the fact, however, that the medicine in its present intensity unfolds also its other symptoms which annul the similarity, it produces a dissimilar chronic disease instead of the former, and, indeed, a more severe and troublesome one, without thereby extinguishing the old original one.

This will be decided in the first sixteen, eighteen or twenty days of the action of the medicine which has been given in too large a dose, and it must then be checked, either by prescribing its antidote, or, if this is not as yet known, by giving another antipsoric medicine fitting as well as possible, and indeed in *a very moderate dose*, and if this does not suffice to extinguish this injurious medicinal disease, another still should be given as homœopathically suitable as possible.*

Now when the stormy assault caused by too large a dose of medicine, although homœopathically selected, has been assuaged through an antidote or the later use of some other antipsoric remedies, then, later on, the same antipsoric remedy—which had been hurtful only because of its over-large dose—can be used again, and, indeed, as soon as it is homœopathically indicated, with the greatest success, only in a *far* smaller dose and in a *much* more highly potentized attenuation, *i. e.*, in a milder quality.

The physician can, indeed, make no worse mistake than *first*, to consider as too small the doses which I (forced by experience) have reduced after manifold trials and which are indicated with every antipsoric remedy and *secondly*, the wrong choice of a remedy, and *thirdly*, the hastiness which does not allow each dose to act its full time.

The first error I have already spoken of, and would only add that nothing is lost if the dose is given even smaller than I have prescribed. *It can hardly be given too small*, if only everything in the diet and the remaining mode of life of the patient which would obstruct or counteract the action of the medicine is avoided. The

---

*I have myself experienced this accident, which is very obstructive to a cure and cannot be avoided too carefully. Still ignorant of the strength of its medicinal power, I gave *Sepia* in too large a dose. This trouble was still more manifest when I gave *Lycopodium* and *Silicea*, potentized to the one-billionth degree, giving four to six pellets, though only as large as poppy seeds. *Discite moniti!*

medicine will still produce all the good effects which can at all be expected from a medicine, if only the antipsoric was homœopathically, correctly selected according to the carefully investigated symptoms of the disease, and if the patient does not disturb its effects by his violation of the rules. If ever it should happen that the choice has not been correctly made, *the great advantage remains that the incorrectly selected medicine in this smallest dose may, in the manner indicated above, be counteracted more easily*, whereupon the cure may be continued without delay with a more suitable antipsoric.

As to the *second* chief error in the cure of chronic diseases (*the unhomœopathic choice of the medicine*) the homœopathic beginner (many, I am sorry to say, remain such beginners their life long) sins chiefly through inexactness, lack of earnestness and through love of ease.

With the great conscientiousness which should be shown in the restoration of a human life endangered by sickness, more than in anything else, the homœopath, if he would act in a manner worthy of his calling, should investigate first the whole state of the patient, the internal cause as far as it is remembered, and the cause of the continuance of the ailment, his mode of life, his quality as to mind, soul and body, together with all his symptoms (see directions in *Organon*), and then he should carefully find out in the work on Chronic Diseases, as well as in the work on Materia Medica Pura, a remedy covering in similarity, as far as possible, all the moments, or at least the most striking and peculiar ones, with its own peculiar symptoms; and for this purpose he should not be satisfied with any of the existing repertories—a carelessness only too frequent; for these books are only intended to give light hints as to one or another remedy that might be selected, but they can never dispense him from making the research at the first fountain heads. He who does not take the trouble of treading this path in all critical and complicated diseases, and, indeed, with all patience and intelligence, but contents himself with the vague hints of the repertories in the choice of a remedy, and who thus quickly dispatches one patient after the other, does not deserve the honorable title of a genuine homœopath, but is rather to be called a bungler, who on that account has continually to change his remedies until the patient loses patience; and, as his ailments have, of course, only been aggravated, he must leave this aggravator of diseases, whereby the art itself suffers discredit instead of the unworthy disciple of art.

This disgraceful love of ease (in the calling which demands the most conscientious care) often induces such would-be homœopaths to give their medicines merely from the (often problematic) statement of their use (*ab usu in morbis*) which are enumerated in the introductions to the medicines, a method which is altogether faulty and strongly savors of allopathy, as these statements usually only give a few symptoms. They should only serve as a confirmation of a choice made according to the pure actions of the medicines, but never to determine the selection of a remedy, which can cure only when used according to the exact similitude of its homœopathic symptoms. There are, we are sorry to say, even authors who advise following this empiric pathway of error!

The *third* leading mistake which the homœopathic physician cannot too carefully nor too steadfastly avoid while treating chronic diseases is in hastily and thoughtlessly—when a properly moderate dose of a well selected antipsoric medicine has been serviceable for several days—giving some other medicine in the mistaken supposition that so small a dose could not possibly operate and be of use more than eight or ten days. This notion is sought to be supported by the statement that on some day or other, while allowed to continue its action, the morbid symptoms, which were to be eradicated, had shown themselves somewhat from time to time.

But if once a medicine, because it was selected in a correct homœopathic manner, is acting well and usefully, which is seen by the eighth or tenth day, then an hour or even half a day may come when a moderate homœopathic aggravation again takes place. The good results will not fail to appear, but may, in very tedious ailments, not show themselves in their best light before the twenty-fourth or thirtieth day. The dose will then probably have exhausted its favorable action about the fortieth or fiftieth day, and before that time it would be injudicious and an obstruction to the progress of the cure to give any other medicine. Let it not be thought, however, that we should scarcely wait for the time assigned as the probable duration of action to elapse before giving another antipsoric medicine, *that we should hasten to change to a new medicine in order to finish the cure more quickly.* Experience contradicts this notion entirely and teaches on the contrary, that a cure cannot be accomplished more quickly and surely than by allowing the suitable antipsoric to continue its action *so long as the improvement continues*, even if this should be several, yea, *many** days beyond the assigned, supposed time of its duration, so as to delay as long as practicable the giving of a new medicine.

Whoever can restrain his impatience as to this point will reach his object the more surely and the more certainly. Only when the old symptoms, which had been eradicated or very much diminished by the last and the preceding medicines, commence to rise again for a few days, or to be again perceptibly aggravated, then the time has most surely come when a dose of the medicine most homœopathically fitting should be given. Experience and careful observation alone can decide, and it always has decided in my manifold, exact observations so as to leave no doubt remaining.

Now, if we consider the great changes which must be effected by the medicine in the many, variously composite and incredibly delicate parts of our living organism before a chronic miasm so deeply inrooted and, as it were, parasitically interwoven with the economy of our life as psora is, can be eradicated and health

---

*In a case where *Sepia* had showed itself completely homœopathically antipsoric for a peculiar headache that appeared in repeated attacks, and where the ailment had been diminished both as to intensity and duration, while the pauses between the attacks had also been much lengthened, when the attacks re-appeared I repeated the dose, which then caused the attacks to cease for one hundred days (consequently its action continued that long), when it re-appeared to some degree, which necessitated another dose, after which no other attack took place for, now, seven years, while the health was also otherwise perfect.

be thus restored, then it may well be seen how natural it is that, during the long-continued action of a dose of antipsoric medicine, selected homœopathically, assaults may be made by it at various periods on the organism, as it were in undulating fluctuations during this long-continued disease. Experience shows that when for several days there has been an improvement, half-hours or whole hours or several hours will again appear when the case seems to become worse; but these periods, so long as only the original ailments are renewed and no new, severe symptoms present themselves, only show a continuing improvement, being homœopathic aggravations, which do not hinder but advance the cure, as they are only renewed beneficent assaults* on the disease, though they are wont to appear at times sixteen, twenty or twenty-four days after taking a dose of antipsoric medicine.

As a rule, therefore, the antipsoric medicine in chronic diseases continue their action the longer, the more tedious the diseases are. But *vice versa* also those medicines which in the healthy body show a long period of action act only a short time and quickly in acute diseases which speedily run their course (*e. g.*, Belladonna, Sulphur, Arsenic, etc.), and their periods of action are shorter, the more acute the diseases. The physician must, therefore, in chronic diseases allow all antipsoric remedies to act thirty, forty or even fifty

---

*These attacks, however, if the antipsoric remedy was selected fittingly and homœopathically and the dose was a moderate one, during its continued action take place, ever more and more rarely and more feebly; but if the doses were too strong, they come more frequently and more strongly, to the detriment of the patient.

and more days *by themselves*, so long as they continue to improve the diseased state perceptibly to the acute observer, even though gradually; for so long the good effects continue with the indicated doses and these must not be disturbed and checked by any new remedy.*

---

*The importance of avoiding the above-described two errors will hardly be realized by physicians. These great, pure truths will be questioned yet for years, even by most of the homœopathic physicians, and will not, therefore, be practiced, on account of the theoretical reflection and the reigning thought: "It requires quite an effort to believe that so little a thing, so prodigiously small a dose of medicine, could effect the least thing in the human body, especially in coping with such enormously great, tedious diseases; but that the physician must cease to reason, if he should believe that these prodigiously small doses can act not only two or three days, but even twenty, thirty and forty days, and longer yet, and cause, even to the last day of their operation, important, beneficent effects otherwise unattainable." Nevertheless this true theorem is not to be reckoned among those which should be comprehended, nor among those for which I ask a blind faith. I demand no faith at all, and do not demand that anybody should comprehend it. Neither do I comprehend it; it is enough that it is a fact and nothing else. Experience alone declares it, and I believe more in experience than in my own intelligence. But who will arrogate to himself the power of weighing the invisible forces that have hitherto been concealed in the inner bosom of nature when they are brought out of the crude state of apparently dead matter through a new, hitherto undiscovered agency, such as is potentizing by long continued trituration and succussion. But he who will not allow himself to be convinced of this, and who will not, therefore, imitate what I now teach after many years' trial and experience (and what does the physician risk if he imitates it exactly?), *he who is not willing to imitate it exactly* can leave this greatest problem of our art unsolved, *he can also leave the most important chronic diseases uncured*, as they have remained unhealed, indeed, up to the time of my teaching. I have no more to say about this. It seemed

But if these appropriately selected antipsoric medicines are not allowed to act their full time, when they are acting well, the whole treatment will amount to nothing. Another antipsoric remedy which may be ever so useful, but is prescribed too early and before the cessation of the action of the present remedy, or a new dose of the same remedy which is still usefully acting, can in no case replace the good effect which has been lost through the interruption of the complete action of the preceding remedy, which was acting usefully, and which can hardly be again replaced.

---

to me my duty to publish the great truths to the world that needs them, untroubled as to whether people can compel themselves to follow them exactly or not. If it is not done with exactness, let no one boast to have imitated me, nor expect a good result.

Do we refuse to imitate any operation until the wonderful forces of nature on which the result is based are clearly brought before our eyes and made comprehensible even to a child? Would it not be silly to refuse to strike sparks from the stone and flint because we cannot comprehend how so much combined caloric can be in these bodies, or how this can be drawn out by rubbing or striking, so that the particles of steel which are rubbed off by the stroke of the hard stone are melted, and, as glowing little balls, cause the tinder to catch fire? And yet we strike fire with it, without understanding or comprehending this miracle of the inexhaustible caloric hidden in the cold steel, or the possibility of calling it out with a frictional stroke. Again, it would be just as silly as if we should refuse to learn to write because we cannot comprehend how one man can communicate his thought to another through pen, ink and paper—and yet we communicate our thoughts to a friend in a letter without either being able or desirous of comprehending this psychico-physical miracle! Why, then, should we hesitate to conquer and heal the bitterest foes of the life of our fellow-men, the chronic diseases, in the stated way, which, punctually followed, is the best possible method, because we do not see how these cures are effected?

It is a *fundamental rule* in the treatment of chronic diseases: *To let the action of the remedy, selected in a mode homœopathically appropriate to the case of disease which has been carefully investigated as to its symptoms, come to an undisturbed conclusion, so long as it visibly advances the cure and the while improvement still perceptibly progresses.* This method forbids any new prescription, any interruption by another medicine and forbids as well *the immediate repetition of the same remedy.* Nor can there be anything more desirable for the physician than to see the improvement of the patient proceed to its completion unhindered and perceptibly. There are not a few cases, where the practiced careful homœopath sees a single dose of his remedy, selected so as to be perfectly homœopathic, even in a very severe chronic disease, continue uninterruptedly to diminish the ailment for several weeks, yea, months, up to recovery; a thing which could not have been expected better in any other way, and could not have been effected by treating with several doses or with several medicines. To make the possibility of this process in some way intelligible, we may assume, what is not very unlikely, that an antipsoric remedy selected most accurately according to homœopathic principles, even in the smallest dose of a high or the highest potency, can manifest so long-continued a curative force, and at last cure, probably, only *by means of a certain infection* with a very similar medicinal disease which overpowers the original disease, by the process of nature itself, according to which (*Organon*, § 45, Fifth Edition), two diseases which are different, indeed, in their kind but very similar in their manifestations and effects, as also in the ailments and symptoms caused by it, when they meet together in the organism, the stronger disease (which is always the one caused by the medicine, § 33, ibid.) destroys the weaker (the natural one). In this case every new medicine and also a new dose of the same medicine, would interrupt the work of improvement and cause new ailments, an interference which often cannot be repaired for a long time.

But if any unfavorable effects are evolved by the present dose of medicine, *i. e.*, troublesome symptoms which do not belong to this disease, and if the mind of the patient becomes depressed, if only a little at first, still increasingly, then the next dose of the same medicine, given immediately after the former, cannot but become injurious to the patient. Yet when a sudden great and striking improvement of a tedious great ailment follows immediately on the first dose of a medicine, there justly arises much suspicion that the remedy has only acted palliatively, and therefore must never be given again, even after the intervention of several other remedies.

Nevertheless there are cases which make an *exception* to the rule, but which not every beginner should risk finding out.*

---

* Still there has been of late much abuse of this immediate repetition of doses of the same medicine, because young Homœopaths thought it more convenient to repeat, without examination, a medicine which in the beginning had been found to be homœopathically suitable, and which had, therefore, in the beginning, proved serviceable, and even to repeat it frequently without examination, so as to heal more quickly.

The only allowable *exception* for an *immediate repetition of the same medicine* is when the dose of a well-selected and in every way suitable and beneficial remedy has made some beginning toward an improvement, but its action ceases too quickly, its power is too soon exhausted, and the cure does not proceed any further. This is rare in chronic diseases, but in acute diseases and in chronic diseases that rise into an acute state it is frequently the case. It is only then,—as a practiced observer may recognize—*when the peculiar symptoms of the disease to be treated, after fourteen, ten, seven, and even fewer days, visibly cease to diminish, so that the improvement manifestly has come to a stop, without any disturbance of the mind and without the appearance of any new troublesome symptoms, so that the former medicine would still be perfectly homœopathically suitable*, only then, I say, is it useful, and probably necessary to give a dose of the same medicine of a similarly small amount, but most safely in a different degree of dynamic potency.* When the remedy is

---

We may declare at once, that the practice of late, which has even been recommended in public journals, of giving the patient several doses of the same medicine to take with him, so that he may take them himself at certain intervals, without considering whether this repetition may affect him injuriously, seems to show a negligent empiricism, and to be unworthy of a homœopathic physician, who should not allow a new dose of a medicine to be taken or given without convincing himself in every case beforehand as to its usefulness.

*If it, *e. g.*, has first been given in the 30th potency, it will now be given in perhaps the 18th, and if a repetition should be again found serviceable and necessary, it might afterwards be given in the 24th, and later perhaps also in the 12th and 6th, etc., if, *e. g.*,

thus modified, the vital force of the patient will allow itself more easily to be further affected by the same medicine, so as to effect by it everything that may be expected of this medicine and in this ailment.*

To adduce an example: a freshly arisen eruption of itch belongs to those diseases which might soonest permit the repetition of the dose (Sulphur), and which does permit it the more frequently, the sooner after the infection the itch is received for treatment, as it then approaches the nature of an acute disorder, and demands its remedies in more frequent doses than when it has been standing on the skin for some time. But this repetition should be permitted only when the preceding dose has largely exhausted its action (after six, eight or ten days), and the dose should be just as small as the preceding one, and be given in a different potency. Nevertheless it is in such a case often serviceable, in answer to a slight change of symptoms, to interpose between the doses of pure Sulphur, a small dose of *Hepar sulphuris calcareum.* This also should

---

the chronic disease should have taken on itself an acute character. A dose of medicine may also have been suddenly counteracted and annihilated by a grave error in the regimen of the patient, when perhaps a dose of the former serviceable medicine might again be given with the modification mentioned above.

*In cases where the physician is certain as to the homœopathic specific to be used, the first attenuated dose may also be dissolved in about four ounces of water by stirring it, and one-third may be drunk at once, and the second and third portions on the following days; but it should each time be again stirred so as to increase the potency and thus to change it. Thereby the remedy seems to take a deeper hold on the organism and hasten the restoration in patients who are vigorous and not too sensitive.

be given in various potencies, if several doses should be needed from time to time. Often, also, according to circumstances, a dose of Nux vomica (x) or one of Mercury (x)* may be used between.

If I except Sulphur, Hepar sulphuris and in some cases Sepia, the other antipsoric remedies can seldom be usefully given in immediately repeated doses. Indeed it is hardly ever needed in chronic diseases, as we have a goodly supply of antipsoric remedies at our disposal, so that as soon as one well selected remedy has completed its action, and a change of symptoms, *i. e.*, a change in the total image of the disease, appears, another antipsoric remedy homœopathically appropriate to the altered case may be chosen to greater advantage and with a more sure prospect of hastening the cure, than if we take the risk of prescribing the former medicine which now is no longer altogether adequate. Nevertheless in very tedious and complex cases, which are mostly such as have been mismanaged by allopathic treatment, it is nearly always necessary to give again from time to time during the treatment, a dose of Sulphur or of Hepar (according to the symptoms), even to the patients who have been before dosed with large allopathic doses of Sulphur and with sulphur-baths; but then only after a previous dose of Mercury (x).

Where, as is usually the case in chronic diseases, various antipsoric remedies are necessary, the more frequent sudden change of them is a sign that the phy-

* That the itch-patient during such a treatment must avoid every external application, however harmless it may appear, *e. g.*, the washing with black soap is not necessary to emphasize.

sician has selected neither the one nor the other in an appropriately homœopathic manner, and had not properly investigated the leading symptoms of the case before prescribing a new remedy. This is a frequent fault into which the homœopathic physician falls in urgent cases of chronic diseases, but oftener still in acute diseases from overhaste, especially when the patient is a person very dear to his heart. I cannot too urgently warn against this fault.

Then the patient naturally falls into such an irritated state that, as we say, no medicine acts, or shows its effect,* yea, so that the power of response in the patient is in danger of flaring up and expiring at the least further dose of medicine. In such a case no further benefit can be had through medicine, but there may be in use a calming mesmeric stroke made from the crown of the head (on which both the extended hands should rest for about a minute) slowly down over the body, passing over the throat, shoulders, arms, hands, knees and legs down over the feet and toes. This may be repeated if necessary.

A dose of homœopathic medicine may also be moderated and softened by allowing the patient to smell† a small pellet moistened with the selected

---

* That a homœopathically potentized dose of medicine should ever fail of having an effect in a treatment conducted *with care*, I think impossible; I have never experienced it.

† Even persons born without the sense of smell or who have lost it through disease, may expect equally efficient help from drawing in the imperceptible vapor (proceeding from the medicine and contained in the vial) through one nostril or the other, as those do who are gifted with the sense of smell. From this it follows that the nerves possessing merely the sense of touch receive the

remedy in a high potency, and placed in a vial the mouth of which is held to the nostril of the patient, who draws in only a momentary little whiff of it. By such an inhalation the powers of any potentized medicine may be communicated to the patient in any degree of strength. One or more such medicated pellets, and even those of a larger size, may be in the smelling-bottle, and by allowing the patient to take longer or stronger whiffs, the dose may be increased a hundred fold as compared with the smallest first mentioned. The period of action of the power of a potentized medicine taken in by such inhalation and spread over so large a surface (as that of the nostrils and of the lungs) lasts as long as that of a small massive dose taken through the mouth and the fauces.

Such medicated pellets kept in a stoppered vial retain their medicinal power quite undiminished, even if the vial be opened a number of times in many years for the purpose of inhalation; *i. e.*, if the vial be preserved from sunshine and heat. This method of allowing the patient to be acted upon by smelling the potentized medicine has great advantages in the manifold mishaps which often obstruct and interrupt the treatment of chronic diseases. The antidote to remove these mishaps as quickly as possible the patient may also best receive in greater or less strength through inhalation, which acts most quickly on the nerves and so also affords the most prompt assistance, by which also the continuation of the treatment of the chronic disease is least delayed. When the mishap

salutary impression and communicate it unfailingly to the whole nervous system.

has thus been obviated most speedily, the antipsoric medicine before taken frequently continues its interrupted action for some time. But the dose of the inhaled medicine must be so apportioned to the morbid interruption that its effect just suffices to extinguish the disadvantage arising from the mishap, without going any deeper or being able to continue its operation any further.

If a homœopathic physician, scrupulous at the wrong occasion, should ask me how he might fill up the many days after giving a dose, so that it may continue its action undisturbed during the above-mentioned long time, and so satisfy, without injuring, the patient who every day* asks for this medicine, I reply with two

*No old established custom among the people, be it ever so hurtful, can be suddenly changed. So also the homœopathic physician cannot avoid allowing a new chronic patient to take at least one little powder a day; the difference between this and the many medicinal doses of allopaths is still very great. During this daily taking of a powder, following the numbers, it will be a great benefit to the poor patient who is often intimidated by slanderers of the better medical art, if he does not know whether there is a dose of medicine in every powder, nor again, in which one of them? If he knew the latter and should know, that to-day's number contains the medicine of which he expects so much, his fancy would often play him an evil trick, and he would imagine that he feels sensations and changes in his body, which do not exist; he would note imaginary symptoms and live in a continual inquietude of mind; but if he daily takes a dose, and daily notices no evil assault on his health, he become more equable in disposition (being taught by experience), expects no ill effects, and will then quietly note the changes in his state which are actually present, and therefore can only report the truth to his physician. On this account it is best that he should daily take his powder, without knowing whether there is medicine in all or in a certain powder; thus he

words, that he should be given every day at the usual time for medicine a dose of sugar of milk, about three grains, which shall be marked as usual with continuous numbers.* I remark here, that I consider the sugar of milk thus used as an invaluable gift of God.†

We cannot flatter ourselves that the antipsoric medicine given was rightly selected, or that it will

---

will not expect more from to-day's powder than from yesterday's or that of the day before.

*Chronic patients who firmly trust in the honesty and skill of their physician will be satisfied, without any afterthoughts, to receive such a dose of sugar of milk every two, four or seven days, according to the disposition of each, and nevertheless retain a firm confidence, as, indeed, is only just and reasonable.

†There were some anxious purists, who were afraid that even the pure sugar of milk, either in itself or changed by long trituration, might have medicinal effects. But this is a vain, utterly unfounded fear, as I have determined by very exact experiments. We may use the crude, pure sugar of milk as a food, and partake of considerable quantities of it, without any change in the health, and so also the triturated sugar. But to destroy at the same time the fear to which utterance has been given by some hypochondriacs, that through a long trituration of the sugar of milk alone, or in the potentizing of medicines, something might rub off from the porcelain mortar (silica), which being potentized by this same trituration would be bound to become strongly acting Silicea ($_1$), I took a new porcelain triturating bowl in which the glazing had been rubbed off, with a new porcelain pestle, and had one hundred grains of pure sugar of milk, divided into portions of thirty-three grains, triturated eighteen times for six minutes at a time and as frequently scraped for four minutes with a porcelain spatula, in order to develop by this three hours' strong trituration a medicinal power either of the sugar of milk or of the silica or of both; but my preparation remained as indifferent and unmedicinal as the crude, merely nutritive sugar of milk, of which I convinced myself by experiments on very sensitive persons.

forward the cure of a chronic disease, if it quickly and entirely destroys as if by a stroke of magic the most troublesome symptoms, old, great, continuous pains, tonic or clonic spasms, etc., so that the patient almost immediately after taking the medicine, fancies himself as much freed from sufferings as if he were already restored, and as if in heaven. This deceptive effect shows that the medicine here acts enantiopathically as an opposite or palliative, and that in the days following we cannot expect anything from this remedy but an aggravation of the original disease. As soon then as this deceptive improvement within a few days begins again to turn to aggravation, it is high time to give either the antidote to this medicine, or, when this cannot be had, a medicine which is homœopathically more appropriate. Very rarely will such an enantiopathic remedy do any good in the future. If the medicine which is thus antipathic at once in the beginning, *i. e.*, which seemed so to alleviate, is inclined to reciprocal action, it is possible that when the aggravation from this dose takes place, a second dose of the same remedy may produce the contrary, and thus bring about a lasting improvement, as I have at least perceived in Ignatia.

In such cases we may also successfully use, for the ailments following after a few days from such an antipathic remedy, one of the remaining medicines from the considerable store laid down in *Materia Medica Pura*, in the "*Arckiv der homœopathischen Heilkunst*" or in "*Annalen.*" This may be done for a few days until the Psora-disease returns to its customary routine course, when a homœopathically selected antipsoric medicine is to be given to continue the cure.

Among the mishaps which disturb the treatment only in a temporary way, I enumerate: overloading the stomach (this may be remedied by hunger, *i. e.*, by only taking a little thin soup instead of the meal and a little coffee); disorder of the stomach from fat meat, especially from eating pork (to be cured by fasting and *pulsatilla*); a disorder of the stomach which causes rising from the stomach after eating and especially nausea and inclination to vomit (by highly potentized *antimonium crudum*); taking cold in the stomach by eating fruit (by smelling of *arsenicum*); troubles from spirituous liquors (*nux vomica*); disorder of the stomach with gastric fever, chilliness and cold (*bryonia alba*); fright (when the medicine can be given at once, and especially when the fright causes timidity, by *poppy-juice* (*opium*); but if aid can only be rendered later, or when vexation is joined with the fright, by *aconite;* but if sadness is caused by the fright, *ignatia seeds*); vexation which causes anger, violence, heat, irritation, by *chamomilla*, (but if beside the vexation there is chilliness and coldness of the body, by *bryonia*); vexation with indignation, deep internal mortification (attended with throwing away what was held in the hand, by *staphisagria*); indignation with silent internal mortification (by *colocynthis*); unsuccessful love with quiet grief (by *ignatia*); unhappy love with jealousy (by *hyoscyamus*); a severe cold (next to keeping the house or the bed) by *nux vomica;* when diarrhœa resulted, by *dulcamara;* or if followed by pains, *coffea cruda;* or if followed by fever and heat, by *aconite;* a cold which is followed by suffocative fits, (by *ipecacuanha*); colds followed by pains and an inclination to weep, (by *coffea cruda*); cold with consequent coryza and loss of the sense of smell and of taste, (by *pulsatilla*) ; overlifting or strains (sometimes by *arnica*, but most certainly by *rhus toxicodendron*); contusions and wounds inflicted by blunt instruments, (by *arnica*); burning of the skin (by compresses of water mixed with a dilution of highly potentized *arsenicum*, or uninterrupted application for hours of alcohol heated by means of very hot water) ; weakness from loss of fluids and blood, (by *china*); homesickness with redness of the cheeks, (by *capsicum*).

But during the treatment of chronic diseases by antipsoric remedies we often need the other non-antipsoric store of medicines in cases where epidemic diseases or intermediate diseases (*morbi intercurrentes*) arising usually from meteoric and telluric causes attack our chronic patients, and so not only temporarily disturb the treatment, but even *interrupt* it for a longer time. Here the other homœopathic remedies will have to be used, wherefore I shall not enter upon this here, except to say that the antipsoric treatment will have for the time to be totally discontinued, so long as the treatment of the epidemic disease which has also seized our (chronic) patient may last, even if a few weeks in the worst cases may thus be lost. But here also, if the disease is not too severe, the above mentioned method of applying the medicine by smelling a moistened pellet is often sufficient to help, and the cure of the acute disease may thus be extraordinarily shortened.

The intelligent homœopathic physician will soon

note the point of time when his remedies have completed the cure of the epidemic intermediate disease*

---

* Usually these epidemic intermediate diseases appear in the form of a fever (if they are not the permanent miasms, small-pox, measles, dysentery, whooping cough, etc.). There are fevers of various kinds, a continuous acute fever, or a slow remittent, or an intermittent fever. Intermittent fevers appear almost every year in a somewhat changed form. Since I have learned to cure chronic diseases and maladies by a homœopathic extirpation of their psoric source, I have found the epidemically current intermittent fevers almost every year different in their character and in their symptoms, and they therefore require almost every year a different medicine for their specific cure. One year they require arsenicum, another belladonna, another antimonium crudum, or spigelia, aconite, with ipecacuanha, alternating with nux vomica, sal ammoniacum, natrum muriaticum, opium, cina, alone or in alternation with capsicum, or capsicum alone, menyanthes trifoliata, calcarea carbonica, pulsatilla, one of the two carbos, arnica, alone or in alternation with ipecacuanha, and with these they were cured in a few days. I would not, indeed, except any one of the non-antipsoric medicines, if they are only homœopathic to the whole complex of the symptoms of the prevailing fever, in its attack as well as in its apyrexia (see *von Bœnninghausen*, Versuch e. hom. Therapie d. Wechselfiebers, 1833, Muenster), but I would almost always except cinchona; for this can only *suppress its type* in many large doses in a concentrated form (as quinine), and then it changes it into a cachexy of quinine, which it is difficult to cure. (*China* is only appropriate to the *endemic* intermittent fever in marshy regions, and even this can only be rightly cured by it in connection with antipsoric remedies.) Even at the beginning of the treatment of an *epidemic* intermittent fever, the homœopathic physicia is most safe in giving every time an attenuated dose of sulphur or in appropriate cases, hepar sulphuris in a fine little pellet or by means of smelling, and in waiting its effects for a few days, until the improvement resulting from it ceases, and then only he will give, in one or two attenuated doses, the non-antipsoric medicine which has been found homœopathically appropri-

and when the peculiar course of the chronic (psoric) malady is continued.

The symptoms of the original chronic disease will, however, always be found somewhat varied after the cure of such a prevailing intermediate disease. Also another part of the body will be found suffering, so that the homœopathic physician will choose his anti-psoric remedy according to the totality of the remaining symptoms, and not simply give the one he intended to give before the intermediate disease appeared.

When the physician is called to treat such a prevalent disease in a patient whom he had not before attended as a chronic patient he will not infrequently find, especially if the fever was considerable, that after overcoming it by the remedies which had been homœopathically specific with other patients of this kind, the full restoration to health does not follow even with good diet and mode of living: but incidents of another kind will show themselves (usually called after-pains or secondary diseases) and these will gradually be aggravated and threaten to become chronic. Here the homœopathic physician will nearly always have to meet a Psora which is developing into a chronic disease, and this will have to be cured according to the principles here laid down.

Here is a fitting opportunity to note that the great

---

ate to the epidemy of this year. These doses should however only be given at the end of an attack. *With all patients in intermittent fever, psora is essentially involved in every epidemy*, therefore an attenuated dose of sulphur or of hepar sulphuris is necessary at the beginning of every treatment of epidemic intermittent fever, and makes the restoration of the patient more sure and easy.

epidemic diseases: small-pox, measles, purple rash, scarlet fever, whooping cough, fall dysentery and typhoid, when they complete their course, especially without a judicious homœopathic treatment, leave the organism so shaken and irritated, that with many who seem restored, the Psora which was before slumbering and latent now awakes quickly, either into itch-like eruptions* or into other chronic disorders, which then reach a high degree in a short time, if they are not treated properly in an antipsoric manner. This is due to the great exhaustion of the organism which still prevails. The allopathic physician, when such a patient, as is frequently the case, dies after all his unsuitable treatment, declares that he has died from the *sequelæ* of whooping cough, measles, etc.

The *sequelæ* are, however, the innumerable chronic diseases in numberless forms of developed Psora which have hitherto been unknown as to their origin and consequently remained uncured.

Epidemic and sporadic fevers, therefore, as well as the miasmatic acute diseases, if they do not soon terminate and pass directly over into good health (even

---

* When such an eruption appears in any quantity, it is called by writers *scabies spontanea* (spontaneous itch)—a mere chimera and nonentity, for as far as history goes, no itch has arisen except from infection, and it cannot now arise again of itself without infection with the miasma of itch. But this phenomenon after acute fever is nothing else than the secondary eruption so often mentioned above springing from the slumbering and latent Psora remaining within after the repression (or more rarely the gradual disappearance) from the skin of the original eruption of itch. This eruption frequently leaves the skin of itself and it has never been proved that it infected any other person with the itch.

when the epidemic and acute miasmatic part has found a homœopathic specific which has been rightly used against them), often need an antipsoric assistance, which I have usually found in Sulphur, if the patient had not used shortly before a medicine containing Sulphur, in which case another antipsoric suitable to this particular case will have to be used.

Endemic diseases, with their striking pertinacity, depend almost wholly on a psoric complication, or on Psora modified by the peculiarity of the nature of the locality (and the especial mode of life of the inhabitants), so that, *e. g.*, an intermittent fever originating in a marshy region, the patients, even after removal into a dry region, often remain uncured despite all their use of China, unless the antipsoric treatment is especially used. The exhalation from swamps seems to be one of the strongest physical causes of the development of the Psora latent within with so many persons* and this most of all in hot countries. Without an almost regular use of the best antipsoric method of cure, we shall never succeed in removing the murderous qualities of humid climates and changing them into passably healthy, habitable regions. Man may accustom himself to the extreme degrees of atmospheric heat, as well as to the most violent cold, and can live joyous and healthy in both extremes. Why should he not be able to accustom himself to marshy regions just

* Presumably these exhalations possess a quality which as it were paralyzes the vital force of the organism (which in an ordinary state of health is able to keep down the internal Psora which always endeavors to manifest itself) and thus predisposes to putrid and nervous fevers.

as well as to the driest mountain regions, if there were not a hitherto undiscovered and unconquered enemy of vigorous life and lasting health, lying in ambush in marshy regions, *i. e.*, Psora? Wherever Psora lies latent within (and how frequently is this the case?) it is developed into chronic diseases of every kind, especially those in which the liver is most affected, through stagnant water and the gases that emanate from damp soil and from swamps; and this is effected *more surely*, yea, *unavoidably*, by these causes than bv any other physical power injurious to health.

The latest symptoms that have been added to a chronic disease which has been left to itself (and thus has not been aggravated by medical mismanagement) are always the first to yield in an antipsoric treatment; but the oldest ailments and those which have been most constant and unchanged, among which are the constant local ailments, are the last to give way; and this is only effected, when all the remaining disorders have disappeared and the health has been in all other respects almost totally restored. In the general maladies which come in repeated attacks, *e. g.*, the periodic kinds of hysteria, and different kinds of epilepsy, etc., the attacks may quickly be made to cease by a suitable antipsoric; but to make this cessation reliable and lasting, the whole indwelling Psora must be completely cured.

The frequent request of a patient to have one symptom, which above others is troublesome to him, removed first of all, is impracticable, but the ignorant patient should be excused for his request.

In the daily written report during the use of an antipsoric medicine, the patient who lives *at a distance* should underscore once, for the information of the physician, those incident symptoms during the day, which after a considerable time or a long time he has now felt again for the first time; but those which he never had before and which he first felt on that day, he should *underscore twice.* The former symptoms indicate that the antipsoric has taken hold of the root of the evil, and will do much for its thorough cure, but the latter, if they appear more frequently and more strongly, give the physician a hint that the antipsoric was not selected quite homœopathically, and should be interrupted in time and replaced by a more appropriate one.

When the treatment is about half completed, the diminished disease commences to return into the state of latent Psora; the symptoms grow weaker and weaker, and at last the attentive physician will only find traces of it; but he must follow these to their complete disappearance, for the smallest remnant retains a germ for a renewal of the old ailment.* If the physician should here give up the treatment and suppose what the common man (and also the higher class of the non-medical public) is apt to say: "It will now likely get right of itself," a great mistake would be made; for in time there would develop (especially when any important untoward events take place), out of this little remnant of this only diminished Psora, a new chronic disease which gradually would increase

* So from the water-polypus which has several of its branches lopped off, in time new branches will shoot forth.

unavoidably, according to the nature of diseases springing from unextinguished chronic miasms as shown above.

The *cito, tuto et jucunde* (quickly, safely and pleasantly) of Celsus, the patient may reasonably ask from his physician, and from the homœopath he can rightly *expect* this in acute diseases springing from occasional causes, as well as in the well-defined intermediate diseases prevalent at times (the so-called intercurrent diseases).

But with especial regard to the "Cito" (quickly), *i. e.*, the hastening of the cure, the nature of the case forbids it, at least in inveterate chronic ailments.*

The cure of great chronic diseases of ten, twenty, thirty and more years' standing (*if they have not been mismanaged by an excess of allopathic treatments, or indeed, as is often the case, mismanaged into incurableness*) may be said to be quickly annihilated if this is done in one or two years. If with younger, robust persons this takes place in one-half the time, then on the other hand in advanced age, even with the best treatment on the part of the physician and the most punctual observance of rules on the part of the patient and his attendants, considerable time must be added to the usual period of the cure. It will also be found

* Only an ordinary ignorant practitioner can lightly promise to cure a severe inveterate disease in four to six weeks. He need not, indeed, keep his promise! What does he risk, if as a matter of course, his treatment only aggravates the disease? Can he lose anything? Any honor? No; for his colleagues, who are like him, do no better. Can he lose in self-respect? Should he yet have any to lose?

intelligible that such a long-continued (psoric) chronic disease, the original miasm of which has had so much time and opportunity in a long life to insert its parasitical roots as it were, into all the joints of the tender edifice of life, is at last so intimately interwoven with the organism that even with the most appropriate medical treatment, careful mode of life and observance of rules on the part of the patient, great patience and sufficient time will be required to destroy this many armed polypus in all its parts, while sparing the independence of the organism and its powers.

The strength of a patient under an antipsoric treatment, even if it should be continued ever so long, ought continually to increase from the very commencement of the correct treatment even to the restoration of health and of the normal state. The strength increases during the whole of the cure without the use of the so-called tonics, and the patients joyously rise up again of themselves in proportion as their life is delivered from its corroding enemy.*

The best time for taking a dose of antipsoric medicine seems to be, not an hour before going to bed but, rather, early in the morning while fasting. The medicine in the numbered paper† (as also all that succeed),

---

* It is inconceivable how allopathic physicians could think of curing chronic diseases through a continuance of exhausting and debilitating treatments, without being restrained by their lack of success from repeating continually their perverse treatment. The *amara* which they give between, together with the quinine, without being able to supply the strength lost, only add new evils.

† Numbering the powders continuously has the convenience that the physician when the patients render their daily report (espe-

if it is desired that it should act but feebly, should be taken dry and allowed to dissolve on the tongue, or be moistened with two or three drops of water on a spoon, and by itself, without in either case drinking anything after it or eating anything within half an hour or a whole hour.*

After taking the medicine the patient should keep perfectly quiet at least a full hour, but without going to sleep (sleep delays the beginning of the action of the medicine). He must avoid during this hour, as indeed throughout the treatment, all disagreeable excitement, nor should he strain his mind immediately after taking the dose, in any way, either by reading or computing, by writing, or by conversations requiring meditation.

The dose of antipsoric medicine must not be taken by females shortly before their menses are expected, nor during their flow; but the dose can be given, if

---

cially those living at a distance), putting first the date and the number of the powder taken that day, can recognize the day when the patient took his medicine, and can judge of the progress of its action according to the report of the following day.

* If the medicine is to act more strongly it must be stirred in a little more water until dissolved before taking it, and in still more water if it is to act still more strongly, and the physician should order the solution taken a portion at a time. If he orders the solution taken in one or three days it must be stirred up not only the first time, but also the other two times, by which every part thus stirred acquires another somewhat higher degree of potency, and so is received more willingly by the vital force. To direct the use of the same solution for a greater number of days is not advisable, as the water, kept longer, would begin to putrefy. How a dose for smelling may be adapted to all degrees of strength, I have mentioned above.

necessary, four days, *i. e.*, about ninety-six hours after the menses have set in. But in case the menses previously have been premature or too profuse, or two long-lasting, it is often necessary to give on this fourth day a small dose of *Nux vomica* (one very small pellet, moistened with a high dynamization) to be smelled, and then, on the fourth or sixth day following, the antipsoric. But if the female is very sensitive and nervous, she ought, until she comes near her full restoration, to smell such a pellet once about seventy-two hours after the beginning of her menses, notwithstanding her continued antipsoric treatment.*

Pregnancy in all its stages offers so little obstruction to the antipsoric treatment, that this treatment is often most necessary and useful in that condition.†

* In such a morbid state of the menses nothing can be done in the cure of chronic diseases without the intermediate use of Nux vomica, which here specifically reduces to order the disharmony arising in the functions of the nerves from so disorderly a flow of the menses, and so quiets this excessive sensitiveness and irritability, which put an insurmountable obstacle in the way of the curative action of the antipsoric remedies.

† In what more certain way could, *e. g*, the return of miscarriage, which is almost exclusively due to Psora, be prevented, and, indeed, be lastingly prevented, than through a judicious antipsoric treatment before or at least during pregnancy? In what more reliable way could the states of the womb, which are not infrequently dangerous, and sometimes fatal even in a proper presentation of the fœtus and in a natural labor, be moved in advance than by a timely antipsoric treatment during pregnancy? Even the improper presentation of the child has, if not always, still very often its only cause in the psoric sickliness of the mother, and the hydrocephalus and other bodily defects of the child have surely this cause! Only the antipsoric treatment of the sickly wife if not before, at least during pregnancy, can remove in advance the moth-

Most necessary, because the chronic ailments then are more developed. In this state of woman, which is quite a natural one, the symptoms of the internal Psora are often manifested most plainly * on account of the increased sensitiveness of the female body and spirit while in this state; the antipsoric medicine therefore acts more definitely and perceptibly during pregnancy, which gives the hint to the physician to make the doses in these cases as small and in as highly potentized attenuations as possible, and to make his selections in the most homœopathic manner.

Sucklings never receive medicine; the mother or wet-nurse receives the remedy instead, and through their milk it acts on the child very quickly, mildly and beneficially.

The corporeal nature (called the life-preserving principle or vital force) when left to itself, since it is without reason, cannot provide anything better than palliatives in chronic diseases, and in the acute diseases springing thence which cause sudden danger to life, owing to the indwelling Psora. These are the causes

---

er's inability for suckling, as also in suckling prevent the frequent sore breasts, the soreness of the nipples, the frequent inclination to erysipelatous inflammations of the breasts and their abscesses, as well the hemorrhages of the uterus during suckling.

* Nevertheless, the entire opposite frequently takes place, so that the wife who before pregnancy was always sickly, and uninterruptedly complaining, feels in unusual good health during every pregnancy and only during this state. And with such cases this time of pregnancy may very well be made use of for antipsoric treatment, which in such a case is directed against the symptoms of the morbid state before pregnancy, so far as this can be remembered.

of the more frequent secretions and excretions of various kinds taking place of themselves now and then in chronic (psoric) diseases, as *e. g.*, diarrhœas, vomiting, perspiration, suppurations, hemorrhages, etc. All these are attended with only temporary alleviations of the chronic original malady, which owing to the losses of humors and of strength thereby only becomes more and more aggravated.

Allopathy has, so far, not been able to do any more than this toward a genuine cure of the chronic diseases; it could only imitate the unreason in corporeal nature in its palliatives (usually without an equal alleviation and with a greater sacrifice of strength). It caused, therefore, more than the other, a hastening of the general ruin, without being able to contribute anything to the extinction of the original malady. To this class belong all the many, indescribable purgatives, the so-called dissolvents, the venesection, cupping, the applying of leeches now so insanely frequent, the sudorifics, the artificial sores, setons, fontanels, exutories, etc.

God be praised, the homœopathic physician who is acquainted with the means of a radical cure, and who thus through the antipsoric treatment can destroy the chronic disease itself, has so little need of the abovementioned applications, which only hasten dissolution, that he has on the contrary to use all care that the patient may not secretly use some of these appliances, following the old routine, diffused over the whole earth by allopathy. He can never yield to the request of the patient, *e. g.*, that he has become accustomed to being bled so and so many times a year, or to be cupped, or to use purgatives or warm baths, and that he therefore needs them. Such things cannot be permitted.

The homœopathic physician who is a master of his art, and God be praised! there is now a not inconsiderable number of such masters in Homœopathy, never allows a drop of blood to be drawn from his patient; he never needs any such or similar means of weakening the body, for such a course evermore remains the negation of curing. Only journeymen, half homœopaths still, I am sorry to say, use such a *contradictio in adjecto* (*weakening while desiring to cure*).*

Only in the one case, where, as in many chronic diseases, the delay in passing evacuations causes great trouble, he will permit (*in the beginning of the treatment* before the antipsoric medicine has had the time [in its after-effects] to produce improvement in this point) if the stool is not passed for three or four days, a clyster of clean, lukewarm water without the least admixture, also perhaps a second, if an evacuation does not result within a quarter of an hour. Rarely a

---

*This may well be pardoned with journeymen and beginners; but when they assume to boast of this noviceship and declare in public journals and books that the incidental use of blood-letting and leeches is indispensable, yea, that it is more essentially homœopathic, they become ridiculous and are to be pitied as tyros and as laboring under delusion; and their patients also are to be pitied. Is it laziness or a haughty preference for their old (although ruinous) allopathic routine, or is it lack of love for their fellowmen which prevents a deeper entering into true, beneficent Homœopathy and an elevation into the troublesome but correct and useful selection of the remedy homœopathically specific in every case, and into that mastery of Homœopathy now no more rare?

third injection will be needed, after waiting a third quarter of an hour. This help which acts chiefly mechanically by expanding the rectum, is harmless when repeated after three or four days if it is necessary, and, as before mentioned, only at the beginning of the treatment—for the antipsoric medicines, among which, in this respect, Lycopodium next to Sulphur has the pre-eminence, usually soon remove this difficulty.

The inexcusable wasting fontanels the homœopathic physician must not at once suppress, if the patient has had them for some time (often for many years), nor before the antipsoric treatment has already made perceptible progress, but if they can be diminished without totally stopping them, this may safely be done even in the beginning of the treatment.

So also the physician should not at once discontinue the woolen underclothing, which is said to prevent the taking of cold and the recommendation of which is carried very far by the ordinary physicians in default of any real assistance. Though they are a burden to the patient, we should wait until there is a visible improvement effected by the antipsorics which remove the tendency to taking cold, and until the warmer season comes. With patients who are very weakly, he should in the beginning change to cotton shirts which rub and heat the skin less, before requiring the patients to put linen underclothing on their skin.

For many easily perceived reasons, but especially in order that his delicate doses of medicine may not be interfered with in their action, the homœopathic physician cannot in his antipsoric treatment allow the intermediate use of any hitherto customary domestic remedy, no perfumery of any kind, no fragrant extracts, no smelling-salts, no Baldwin tea, or any other herb teas, no peppermint confection, no spiced confections or anise-sugar or stomach drops, or liquors, no Iceland-moss, or spiced chocolate, no spice-drops, tooth-tinctures or tooth-powders of the ordinary kinds, nor any of the other articles of luxury.

So-called warm and hot baths for the sake of cleanliness, to which spoiled patients are usually very much attached, are not to be allowed, as they never fail to disturb the health; nor are they needed, as a quick washing of a part or of the whole of the body with lukewarm soap-water fully serves the purpose without doing any injury.

At the end of these directions for treating chronic diseases, I recommended, in the first edition, the lightest electric sparks as an adjuvant for quickening parts that have been for a long time paralyzed and without sensation, these to be used besides antipsoric treatment. I am sorry for this advice, and take it back, as experience has taught me that this prescription has nowhere been followed strictly, but that larger electric sparks have always been used to the detriment of patients; and yet these larger sparks have been asserted to be very small. I, therefore, now advise against this so easily abused remedy, especially, as we can easily remove this appearance of enantiopathic assistance; for there is an efficient *homœopathic* local assistance for paralyzed parts or such as are without sensation. This is found in cold water* locally applied (at 54° Fahrenheit) from mountain-springs and deep wells; either by pouring on these parts for one, two or three minutes, or by douche-baths over the whole body of one to five minutes duration, more rarely or more frequently, even daily or oftener according to the circumstances, together with the appropriate, internal, antipsoric treatment, sufficient exercise in the open air, and judicious diet.

* Water of this and a lower temperature has the primary power of depriving the parts of the living body partly of sensation and partly of motion, in such cases it therefore gives local homœopathic assistance.

THE MEDICINES.

The medicines which have been found most suitable and excellent in chronic diseases so far, I shall present in the following part according to their pure action on the human body, as well those used in the treatment of the diseases of psoric origin, as those used in syphilis and in the figwart-disease.

That we need far fewer remedies to combat the latter than the Psora can not with any thinking man form an argument against the chronic miasmatic nature of the latter and still less against the fact that it is the common source of the other chronic diseases.

The Psora, a most ancient miasmatic disease, in propagating itself for many thousands of years through several millions of human organisms, of which each one had its own peculiar constitution and was exposed to very varied influences, was able to modify itself to such a degree as to cause that incredible variety of ailments which we see in the innumerable chronic patients, with whom the external symptom (which acts vicariously for the internal malady), *i. e.*, the more or less extensive eruption of itch, has been driven away from the skin by a fatal art, or in whom it has disappeared of itself from the skin through some other violent incident.

Hence it seems to have come to pass that this half-spiritual miasma, which like a parasite seeks to inroot its hostile life in the human organism and to continue its life there, could develop itself in so many ways in the many thousands of years, so that it has even caused to spring forth and has born modified offshoots with characteristic properties, which do not indeed deny their descent from their stock (the common Psora), but, nevertheless, differ from one another considerably by some peculiarities. These changes are due in some part to the varying physical peculiarities and climatic differences of the dwelling-places of men afflicted with the Psora,* and in part are moulded by their varying modes of life, *e. g.* children in corrupt city air develop rhachitis, *spina ventosa*, *softening of the bones*, *curvatures*, *cancer of the bones*, *tinea capitis*, scrofula, ringworm; adults exhibit nervous debility, nervous irritability, gout of the joints, etc. And so also the other great varieties in the mode of living and in the occupations of men with their inherited bodily constitutions give to the psoric diseases so many modifications, that it may easily be understood, that more numerous and more varied remedies are needed for the extirpation of all these modifications of the Psora (antipsoric remedies).

I have often been asked by what signs a substance may beforehand be recognized as antipsoric? But

*E. g. the *Sibbens* or *Rade-Syge* commonly found in Norway and in the northwest of Scotland; the *Pellagra* in Lombardy; the *plica polonica* (Koltun, Trichiasis) in Poland and Carinthia, the tumorous leprosy in Surinam; the raspberry-like excrescences (Frambösia) in Guinea called *yaws* and in America *pian;* the exhaustive fever in Hungary called *Tsömör*, the exhausting malady of Virginia (*asthenia Virginensium*), the human degeneration in the deep Alpine villages called *cretin*, the *goitre* in the deep valleys and at their entrances, etc.

there can be no such external visible marks in them; nevertheless while proving several powerful substances as to their pure effects on the healthy body, several of them by the complaints they caused showed me their extraordinary and manifest suitableness for homœopathic aid in the symptoms of clearly defined psoric diseases. Some traces of their qualities leading in this direction gave me in advance some hint as to their probable usefulness; *e. g.* the efficacy of the herb *Lycopodium*, much praised in Poland for the *plica polonica* pointed me to the use of the pollen of lycopodium in similar psoric ailments. The circumstance that some hemorrhages have been arrested by large doses of salt was another hint. So was the usefulness of Guaiacum, Sarsaparilla and Mezereum, even in ancient times where venereal diseases could not be healed by any amount of mercury unless one or the other of these herbs had first removed the Psora complicated with it.

As a rule it was developed from their pure symptoms, that most of the earths, alkalies and acids, as well as the neutral salts composed of them, together with several of the metals, cannot be dispensed with in curing the almost innumerable symptoms of Psora. The similarity in nature of the leading antipsoric, sulphur, to phosphorus and other combustible substances from the vegetable and mineral kingdoms led to the use of the latter, and some animal substances naturally followed them by analogy, in agreement with experience.

Still only those remedies have been acknowledged as antipsoric whose pure effects on the human health gave a clear indication of their homœopathic use in diseases manifestly psoric, confessedly due to infection; so that, with an enlargement of our knowledge of their proper, pure medicinal effects, in time it may be found necessary to include some of our other medicines among the antipsoric remedies; although even now we can with certainty cure, with the antipsorics now recognized, nearly all non-venereal (psoric) chronic diseases, if the patients have not been loaded down and spoiled through allopathic mismanagement with severe medicine-diseases, and when their vital force has not been depressed too low, or very unfavorable external circumstances make the cure impossible. Nevertheless, it need not be specially stated that the other proved, homœopathic medicines, not excepting *Mercury*, cannot be dispensed with in certain states of the psoric diseases.

Homœopathy, by a certain treatment of the crude medicinal substances, which had not been invented before its foundation and development, advances them into the state of progressive and high development of their indwelling forces, in order that it may then use them in curing in the most perfect manner. Some of these medicines in their crude state seem to have a very imperfect, insignificant medicinal action (*e. g.*, common salt and the pollen of Lycopodium). Others (*e. g.*, Gold, Quartz, Alumina) seem to have none at all, but all of them become highly curative by the preparation peculiar to Homœopathy. Other substances, on the other hand, in their crude state are, even in the smallest quantities, so violent in their effects that if they touch the animal fibre, they act upon it in a corroding and destructive manner (*i. g.*, Arsenic and corrosive sublimate) and these medicines are rendered by the same preparation peculiar to Homœopathy not only mild in their effects, but also incredibly developed in their medicinal powers.

The changes which take place in material substances, especially in medicinal ones, through long-continued trituration with a non-medicinal powder, or when dissolved, through a long-continued shaking with a non-medicinal fluid, are so incredible, that they approach the miraculous, and it is a cause of joy that the discovery of these wonderful changes belongs to Homœopathy.

Not only, as shown elsewhere, do these medicinal substances thereby develop their powers in a prodigious degree, but they also change their physico-chemical demeanor in such a way, that if no one before could ever perceive in their crude form any solubility in alcohol or water, after this peculiar transmutation they become wholly soluble in water as well as in alcohol—a discovery invaluable to the healing art.

The brown-black juice of the marine animal *Sepia*, which was formerly only used for drawing and painting, is in its crude state soluble only in water, not in alcohol; but by such a trituration it becomes soluble also in alcohol.

The yellow Petroleum only allows something to be extracted from it through alcohol when it is adulterated with ethereal vegetable oil; but in its pure state while crude it is soluble neither in water nor in alcohol (nor in ether). By trituration it becomes soluble in both substances.

So also the *Pollen of Lycopodium* floats on alcohol and on water, without either of them showing any action upon it—the crude Lycopodium is tasteless and inactive when it enters the human stomach; but when changed in a similar manner through trituration it is not only perfectly soluble in either fluid, but has also developed such extraordinary medicinal powers, that great care must be taken in its medicinal use.

Who ever found marble or oyster-shells soluble in pure water or in alcohol? But this mild *Lime* becomes perfectly soluble in either, by means of this mode of preparation; the same is the case with *Baryta* and *Magnesia* and these substances then exhibit astonishing medicinal powers.

Least of all will anyone ascribe solubility in water and alcohol to quartz, to rock-crystal (many crystals of which have contained enclosed in them drops of water for thousands of years unchanged), or to sand; nor would anyone ascribe to them medicinal power, and yet by the dynamization (potentizing)* peculiar to Homœopathy, by melting silica with an alkaline salt, and then precipitating it from this glass, it not only becomes soluble without any residuum in water and in alcohol, but also then shows prodigious medicinal powers.

---

* In its crude condition and without this preparation quartz and pebbles do not seem to allow a development of their medicinal powers by trituration and therefore it is that the triturating of various m dicines with the indifferent sugar of milk in the porcelain triturating bowl seems to impart to them no admixture of *Silicea* as some anxious purists have vainly feared.

What can I say of the pure metals and of their sulphurets, but that all of them, without any exception become by this treatment equally soluble in water and in alcohol, and every one of them develops the medicinal virtue peculiar to it in the purest, simplest manner and in an incredibly high degree?

But the chemical medicinal substances thus prepared now also stand above the *chemical* laws.

A dose of Phosphorus, potentized highly in a similar manner, may lie in its paper envelope in the desk, and, nevertheless, when taken after a whole year's interval, it will still show its full medicinal power; not that of the Phosphoric acid, but that of the unchanged, uncombined Phosphorus itself. So that no neutralization takes place in this its elevated, and as it were, glorified state.

The medicinal effects of Natrum carbonicum, of Ammonium carbonicum, of Baryta, of Lime, and of Magnesia, in this highly potentized state, when a dose of one of them has been taken, is not neutralized like basic substances taken in a crude form by a drop of vinegar taken afterwards; their medicinal effect being neither changed nor destroyed.

Nitric acid, when thus given in its highly potentized state in which it is serviceable for homœopathic medicinal use, is not changed by a little crude lime or crude soda given after it, as to its strong well defined medicinal action; therefore it is not neutralized.

In this *preparation*, peculiar to Homœopatny, we take one grain in powder of any of the substances treated of in the volumes of the Materia Medica Pura,*

---

* Vegetable substances which can only be procured dry, *e. g*

and especially those of the antipsoric substances* following below, *i. e.*, of silica. carbonate of baryta, carbonate of lime, carbonate of soda and sal ammoniac, carbonate of magnesia, vegetable charcoal, animal charcoal, graphites, sulphur, crude antimony, metallic antimony, gold, platina, iron, zinc, copper, silver, tin. The lumps of the metals which have not yet been

---

cinchona bark, ipecacuanha, etc., are prepared by the same kind of trituration and will completely dissolve when potentized a million fold, not less, with their peculiar powers, in water and alcohol, and may then be preserved as medicines far more easily than the easily spoiled alcoholic tinctures. Of the juiceless vegetable substances, such as oleander, thuja, the bark of mezereum, etc., we may, without making a mistake, take of each about one and a half grains of the fresh leaves, bark, root, etc., without any further preparation, and triturate the same three times with 100 grains of sugar of milk to the millionfold powder trituration. A grain of this dissolved in alcohol and water may be developed in the diluting vials with alcohol to the necessary degree of potency of their powers by giving for each potency two succussive strokes. Also with the freshly expressed juices of the herbs it is best to at once put one drop of the same with as much sugar of milk as is taken for the preparation of the other medicines, so as to triturate it to the millionfold powder attenuation, and then a grain of this attenuation is dissolved in equal parts of water and alcohol, and must be potentized to a further dynamization through the twenty-seven diluting vials by means of two succussive strokes. The fresh juices thus seem to acquire more of dynamization, as experience teaches me, than when the juice without any preparation by triturating is merely diluted in thirty vials of alcohol and potentized each time with two succussive strokes.

* Even phosphorus which is so easily oxidized by exposure to the air is potentized in a similar manner, and thus rendered soluble in these two liquids, and is thus prepared as a homœopathic medicine; but in this case some precautions are used, which will be found below.

beaten out into foil are rubbed off on a fine, hard whetstone under water, some of them, as iron, under alcohol; of mercury in the liquid form one grain is taken, of petroleum one drop instead of a grain, etc. This is first put on about one-third of 100 grains of pulverized sugar of milk, and placed in an unglazed porcelain mortar, or in one from which the glaze has been first rubbed off with wet sand; the medicine and the sugar of milk are then mixed for a moment with a porcelain spatula, and the mixture is triturated with some force for six minutes, the triturated substance is then for four minutes scraped from the mortar and from the porcelain pestle,* which is also unglazed, or has had its glazing rubbed off with wet sand, so that the trituration may be homogeneously mixed. After this has been thus scraped together, it is triturated again without any addition for another six minutes with equal force. After scraping together again from the bottom and the sides for four minutes this triturate (for which the first third of the 100 grains had been used), the second third of the sugar of milk is now added, both are mixed together with the spatula for a moment, triturated again with like force for six min-

* That after the completion of every three hours' trituration of a medicinal substance, the mortar, pestle and spatula are to be several times scalded with boiling water, being after every scalding wiped quite dry and clean, I presuppose as indispensable, so that no idea of spoiling any medicine that may be triturated in it in future may be entertained. If the further precaution is used of exposing mortar, pestle and spatula to a heat approaching red heat, this will dissipate every thought that any least rest of the medicine last triturated can cling to them, and thus even the most scrupulous mind will be satisfied.

utes; then having again scraped the triturate for four minutes, it is triturated a second time (without addition) for six minutes more, and after scraping it together for another four minutes it is mixed with the last third of the powdered sugar of milk by stirring it around with the spatula, and then the whole mixture is again triturated for six minutes, scraped for four minutes, and a second and last time triturated for six minutes; then it is all scraped together and the powder is preserved in a well-stoppered bottle with the name of the substance and the signature 100 because it is potentized one hundred fold.*

---

* Only phosphorus needs some modification in the preparation of the first attenuation to the 100th degree. Here the hundred grains of sugar of milk are at once put into the triturating bowl and, with about twelve drops of water, they are stirred by means of the wet pestle into a thickish pap; one grain of phosphorus is then cut into numerous pieces, say, twelve, and kneaded in with the moist pestle and rather stamped than rubbed into it, while the mass which often clings to the pestle is as often scraped into the mortar. Thus the little crumbs of phosphorus are rubbed to little invisible dust particles in the thick pap of sugar of milk even in the first two periods of six minutes each, without the appearance of the least spark. During the third period of six minutes the stamping may pass over into rubbing, because the mass is then approaching the form of powder. During the succeeding three periods of six minutes each the trituration is carried on only with a moderate force, and after every six minutes the powder is scraped from the mortar and the pestle for several minutes, which is done easily, as this powder does not adhere tenaciously. After the sixth period of trituration the powder, when standing exposed to the air in the dark, is only feebly luminous, and has but a slight odor. It is put into a well stoppered vial and marked phosphorus $\frac{1}{100}$, the other two triturations $\frac{1}{10000}$, and $\frac{1}{\text{mill.}}$ are prepared like those from other dry medicinal substances.

To potentize the substance to the ten thousandth attenuation, one grain of the powder last mentioned as being the one hundredth is taken with one-third of 100 grains of fresh sugar of milk, stirred in the mortar with a spatula and treated as above, so that every third is triturated twice for six minutes at a time, and after every trituration is scraped together (for about four minutes), before the second third of the sugar of milk is added, and after this has been similarly treated the last third of sugar of milk is stirred into it and again similarly triturated twice for six minutes at a time, when it is scraped together, put in a stoppered vial with the signature $_{10000}$ as it contains the medicine potentized to the ten thousandth attenuation.*

The same is done with one grain of this powder (marked $_{10000}$) in order to bring it to I, and thus to attenuate it to the millionfold potency.

In order to produce a homogeneity in the preparation of the homœopathic and especially the antipsoric remedies, at least in the form of powders, I advise the reducing of medicines only to this millionth potency, no more or no less, and to prepare from this the solutions and the necessary potencies of these solutions; this has been my own custom.

The trituration should be done with force, yet only with so much force that the sugar of milk may not be pressed too firmly to the mortar, but may be scraped up in four minutes.

---

* Thus it will be seen that every attenuation (that to $_{100}$, that to $_{10000}$, and also the third to $_{1000000}$ or I) is prepared by six times triturating for six minutes and six times scraping together for four minutes each time. Thus each one requires one hour.

Now in preparing the solutions * from this, and in bringing the medicines thus potentized one millionfold, into the fluid form, (so that their dynamization may be still further continued), we are aided by the property of *all* medicinal substances, that, when brought to the potency I, they are soluble in water and alcohol; this property is still unknown to chemistry.

The first solution cannot be made in pure alcohol, because sugar of milk will not dissolve in alcohol. The first solution is therefore made in a mixture of half water and half alcohol.

To one grain of the medicinal powder triturated to the millionfold potency I, fifty drops of distilled water are dropped in, and by turning the vial a few times round on its axis it is easily dissolved, when fifty drops of good alcohol † are added, and the vial, which ought only to be filled to two-thirds of its capacity by the mixture, ought to be stoppered and shaken twice, (*i. e.*, with two down-strokes of the arm). It is marked

---

* In the beginning I used to give a small part of a grain of the powders potentized to the $_{\overline{10000}}$ or the I degree by trituration, as a dose. But since *a small part of a grain* is too indefinite a quantity, and since Homœopathy must avoid all indefiniteness and inexactness as much as possible, the discovery that all medicines may be changed from potentized medicinal powders into fluids, with which a definite number of pellets may be moistened for a dose, was of great value to me. From liquids the higher potencies may also be easily prepared.

† For the fifty drops of water as well as for the fifty drops of alcohol a vial containing just that quantity may be used, so that we need not then count the drops, especially as drops of water are not easily counted when it flows from a vial, the mouth of which is not roughened by rubbing with sand.

with the name of the medicine and $_{100\,\mathrm{I}}$.* One drop of this is added to ninety-nine or one hundred drops of pure alcohol, the stoppered vial is then shaken with two strokes of the arm and marked with the name of the medicine and designated $_{10000\,\mathrm{I}}$. One drop of this is added to ninety-nine or one hundred drops of pure alcohol, the corked vial is then shaken with two strokes of the arm and marked with the name of the medicine and $_{\mathrm{II}}$. The preparation of the higher potencies is then continued with two strokes of the arm† every time to the $_{100\,\mathrm{II}}$, $_{10000\,\mathrm{II}}$, etc., but to attain a simple uniformity in practice only the vials with the full numbers $\overline{\mathrm{II}, \mathrm{III}, \mathrm{IV}, \mathrm{V}}$,‡ etc., are used in practice, but

* It will be well to mark on the label that it has been shaken twice, together with the date.

† After many experiments and searching comparisons with the patients I have for several years preferred from conviction to give to the medicinal fluids which are to be elevated to higher potencies and at the same time to be rendered milder, only two shakes (with two strokes of the arm) instead of the ten shakes given by others, because the potentizing in the latter case by the repeated shaking passes far beyond the attenuation at every step (though this is one hundred fold); while yet the end striven for is to develop the medicinal powers only in the degree that the attenuation may reach the end aimed for: to moderate in some degree the strength of the medicine while its power of penetration is increased. The double shake also increases the quantity of the medicinal forces developed, like the tenfold shake, but not in as high a degree as the latter, so that its strength may, nevertheless, be kept down by the one hundred fold attenuation effected, and we thus obtain every time a weaker though somewhat more highly potentized and more penetrating medicine.

‡ Instead of the fractional numbers $\frac{1}{1000000}$ ($\frac{1}{\mathrm{I}}$), $\frac{1}{1000000000000}$ ($\frac{1}{\mathrm{II}}$), etc., these degrees of dynamization are frequently so expressed that only the exponent showing how often one hundred

the intermediate numbers are preserved in boxes or cases with their labels. Thus they will be protected from the effect of daylight.

As the shaking is *only* to take place through *moderate* strokes of the arm, the hand of which holds the vial, it is best to choose the vials just so large that they will be two-thirds fiilled with 100 drops of the attenuated medicine.

Vials that have contained a remedy must never be used for the reception of any other medicine, though they be rinsed ever so often, but new vials must be taken every time.

The pellets which are to be moistened with the medicine should also be selected of the same size, hardly as large as poppy-seeds, made by the confectioner, partly so that the dose may be made small enough, and partly that homœopathic physicians in the preparation of medicines, as also in the giving of doses, may act alike, and thus be able to compare the result of their practice with that of other Homœopaths in the most certain manner.

The moistening of pellets is best done with a quantity, so that a drachm or several drachms of pellets are put into a little dish of stoneware, porcelain or glass; this dish should be more deep than wide, in the form

---

has been multiplied into itself is expressed, thus instead of ^{1}, $_{100}$ $(^{3})$; instead of $\frac{1}{\text{II}}$, $_{100}(^{6})$; instead of ^{1}, $_{100}(^{9})$; instead of $\frac{1}{100}$III $_{100}$ $(^{10})$; instead of $\frac{1}{10000}$IX, $_{100}(^{29})$ and instead of decillion $\frac{1}{\text{X}}$, $_{100}(^{30})$, thus only the exponents as to the third, sixth, ninth, tenth, twenty-ninth and thirtieth potency, etc.

of a large thimble; several drops of the spirituous medicinal fluid should be dropped into it (rather a few drops too many), so that they may penetrate to the bottom and will have moistened all the pellets within a minute. Then the dish is turned over and emptied on a piece of clean double blotting paper, so that the superfluous fluid may be absorbed by it, and when this is done, the pellets are spread on the paper so as to dry quickly. When dry, the pellets are filled in a vial, marked as to its contents, and well stoppered.

All pellets moistened with the spirituous liquid have when dry a dull appearance; the crude, unmoistened pellets look whiter and more shining.

To prepare the pellets to give to patients, one or a couple of such little pellets are put into the open end of a paper capsule containing two or three grains of powdered sugar of milk; this is then stroked with a spatula or the nail of the thumb with some degree of pressure until it is felt that the pellet or pellets are crushed and broken then the pellets will easily dissolve if put into water.

Wherever I mention pellets in giving medicine, I always mean the finest, of the size of poppy-seeds, of which about 200 (more or less) weigh a grain.

The antipsoric medicines treated of in what follows contain no so-called *idiopathic* medicines, since their pure effects, even those of the potentized miasma of itch (*Psorin*) have not been proved enough, by far, that a safe homœopathic use might be made of it. I say *homœopathic* use, for it does not remain *idem* (the same); even if the prepared itch substance should be given to the same patient from whom it was taken, it would not remain *idem* (the same), as it could only be useful to him in a potentized state, since crude itch substance which he has already in his body as an *idem* is without effect on him. But the dynamization or potentizing changes it and modifies it; just as gold leaf after potentizing is no more crude gold leaf inert in the human body, but in every stage of dynamization it is more and more modified and changed.

Thus potentized and modified also, the itch substance (*Psorin*) when taken is no more an *idem* (the same) with the crude original itch substance, but only a *simillimum* (thing most similar). *For between* IDEM *and* SIMILLIMUM *there is no intermediate for any one that can think ;* or in other words between *idem* and *simile* only *simillimum* can be intermediate. Isopathic and *æquale* are equivocal expressions, which if they should signify anything reliable can only signify *simillimum*, because they are not *idem* (ταυτον).

SECOND PART.

ANTIPSORIC MEDICINES.

PREFACE.

CONCERNING THE TECHNICAL PART OF HOMŒOPATHY.[1]

Since I last* addressed the public concerning our healing art, I have had among other things also the opportunity to gain experience as to the best possible mode of administering the doses of the medicines to the patients, and I herewith communicate what I have found best in this respect.

A small pellet of one of the highest dynamizations of a medicine laid dry upon the tongue, or the moderate smelling of an opened vial wherein one or more such pellets are contained, proves itself the smallest and weakest dose with the shortest period of duration in its effects. Still there are numerous patients of so excitable a nature, that they are sufficiently affected by such a dose in slight acute ailments to be cured by it if the remedy is homœopathically selected. Nevertheless the incredible variety among patients as to their irritability, their age, their spiritual and bodily development, their vital power and especially as to the nature of their

---

[1] This preface was prefixed to Vol. III. of the "Chronic Diseases," published in the year 1837.—*Tr.*

* In the beginning of the year 1834 I wrote the first two parts of this work, and although they together contain only thirty-six sheets, my former publisher, Mr. Arnold, in Dresden, took two years to publish these thirty-six sheets. By whom was he thus delayed? My acquaintances can guess that.

disease, necessitates a great variety in their treatment, and also in the administration to them of the doses of medicines. For their diseases may be of various kinds: either a natural and simple one but lately arisen, or it may be a natural and simple one but an old case, or it may be a complicated one (a combination of several miasmata), or again what is the most frequent and worst case, it may have been spoiled by a perverse medical treatment, and loaded down with medicinal diseases.

I can here limit myself only to this latter case, as the other cases cannot be arranged in tabular form for the weak and negligent, but must be left to the accuracy, the industry and the intelligence of able men, who are masters of their art.

Experience has shown me, as it has no doubt also shown to most of my followers, that it is most useful in diseases of any magnitude (not excepting even the most acute, and still more so in the half-acute, in the tedious and most tedious) to give to the patient the powerful homœopathic pellet or pellets only in solution, and this solution in divided doses. In this way we give the medicine, dissolved in seven to twenty tablespoonfuls of water without any addition, in acute and very acute diseases every six, four or two hours; where the danger is urgent, even every hour or every half hour, a tablespoonful at a time; with weak persons or children, only a small part of a tablespoonful (one or two teaspoonfuls or coffeespoonfuls) may be given as a dose.

In chronic diseases I have found it best to give a dose (*e. g.*, a spoonful) of a solution of the suitable medicine at least every two days, more usually every day.

But since water (even distilled water) commences after a few days to spoil, whereby the power of the small quantity of medicine contained is destroyed, the addition of a little alcohol is necessary, or where this is not practicable, or if the patient cannot bear it, I add a few small pieces of hard charcoal to the watery solution. This answers the purpose, except that in the latter case the fluid in a few days receives a blackish tint. This is caused by shaking the liquid, as is necessary every time before giving a dose of medicine, as may be seen below.

Before proceeding, it is important to observe, that our vital principle cannot well bear that the same unchanged dose of medicine be given even twice in succession, much less more frequently to a patient. For by this the good effect of the former dose of medicine is either neutralized in part, or new symptoms proper to the medicine, symptoms which have not before been present in the disease, appear, impeding the cure. Thus even a well selected homœopathic medicine produces ill effects and attains its purpose imperfectly or not at all. Thence come the many contradictions of homœopathic physicians with respect to the repetition of doses.

But in taking one and the same medicine repeatedly (which is *indispensible* to secure the cure of a serious, chronic disease), if the dose is in every case varied and modified only a little in its degree of dynamization, then the vital force of the patient will calmly, and as it were willingly receive *the same* medicine even at brief intervals very many times in succession with the best results, every time increasing the well-being of the patient.

This slight change in the degree of dynamization is even effected, if the bottle which contains the solution of one or more pellets is merely well shaken five or six times, every time before taking it.

Now when the physician has in this way used up the solution of the medicine that had been prepared, if the medicine continues useful, he will take one or two pellets of the same medicine in a lower potency, (*e. g.*, if before he had used the thirtieth dilution, he will now take one or two pellets of the twenty-fourth), and will make a solution in about as many spoonfuls of water, shaking up the bottle, and adding a little alcohol or a few pieces of charcoal. This last solution may then be taken in the same manner, or at longer intervals, perhaps also less of the solution at a time; but every time the solution must be shaken up five or six times. This will be continued so long as the remedy still produces improvement and until new ailments (such as have never yet occurred with other patients in this disease), appear; for in such a case a new remedy will have to be used. On any day when the remedy has produced too strong an action, the dose should be omitted for a day. If the symptoms of the disease alone appear, but are considerably aggravated even during the more moderate use of the medicine, then the time has come to break off in the use of the medicine for one or two weeks, and to await a considerable improvement.*

* In treating acute cases of disease the homœopathic physician

When the medicine has been consumed and it is found necessary to continue the same remedy, if the physician should desire to prepare a new portion of medicine from the same degree of potency, it will be necessary to give to the new solution as many shakes, as the number of shakes given to the last portion amount to when summed up together, and then a few more, before the patient is given the first dose ; but after that, with the subsequent doses, the solution is to be shaken up only five or six times.

In this manner the homœopathic physician will derive all the benefit from a well selected remedy, which can be obtained in any special case of chronic disease by doses given through the mouth.

But if the diseased organism is affected by the physician through this same appropriate remedy at the same time in sensitive spots other than the nerves of

---

will proceed in a similar manner. He will dissolve one (two) pellet of the highly potentized, well selected medicine in seven, ten or fifteen tablespoonfuls of water (without addition) by shaking the bottle. He will then, according as the disease is more or less acute, and more or less dangerous, give the patient every half hour, or every hour, every two, three, four, six hours (after again well shaking the bottle) a whole or a half tablespoonful of the solution, or, in the case of a child, even less. If the physician sees no new symptoms develop, he will continue at these intervals, until the symptoms present at first begin to be aggravated ; then he will give it at longer intervals and less at a time.

As is well known, in cholera the suitable medicine has often to be given at far shorter intervals.

Children are always given these solutions from their usual drinking vessels; a teaspoon for drinking is to them unusual and suspicious, and they will refuse the tasteless liquid at once on that account. A little sugar may be added for their sake.

the mouth and the alimentary canal, *i. e.*, if this same remedy that has been found useful is at the same time in its watery solution rubbed in (even in small quantities) into one or more parts of the body which are most free from the morbid ailments (*e. g.*, on an arm, or on the thigh or leg, which have neither cutaneous eruptions, nor pains, nor cramps)—then the curative effects are *much* increased. The limbs which are thus rubbed with the solution may also be varied, first one, then another. Thus the physician will receive a greater action from the medicine homœpathically suitable to the chronic patient, and can cure him more quickly, than by merely internally administering the remedy.

This mode of procedure has been frequently proved by myself and found extraordinarily curative; yea, attended by the most startling good effects; the medicine taken internally being at the same time rubbed on the skin externally. This procedure will also explain the wonderful cures, of rare occurrence, indeed, where chronic crippled patients *with sound skin* recovered quickly and permanently by a few baths in a mineral water, the medicinal constituents of which were to a great degree homœopathic to their chronic disease.*

---

* On the other hand such baths have also inflicted a proportionally greater injury with patients who suffered from ulcers and cutaneous eruptions; for these were driven by them from the skin, as may be done by other external means, when after a short period of health, the vital force of the patient transferred the internal uncured disease to another part of the body, and one much more important to life and health. Thus, *e. g.*, may be produced the

The limb, therefore, on which the solution is to be rubbed in, must be *free from cutaneous ailments*. In order to introduce also here change and variation, when several of the limbs are free from cutaneous ailments, one limb after the other should be used, in alternation on different days, (best on days when the medicine is not taken internally). A small quantity of the solution should be rubbed in with the hand, until the limb is dry. Also for this purpose, the bot tle should be shaken five or six times.

Convenient as the mode of administering the medicine above described may be, and much as it surely advances the cure of chronic diseases, nevertheless, the greater quantity of alcohol or whiskey or the several lumps of charcoal which have to be added in warmer weather to preserve the watery solution were still objectionable to me with many patients.

I have, therefore, lately found the following mode of administration preferable with careful patients: From a mixture of about five tablespoonfuls of pure water and five tablespoonfuls of French brandy, which is kept on hand in a bottle, 200, 300 or 400 drops (according as the solution is to be weaker or stronger) are dropped into a little vial, which may be half-filled with it, and in which the medicinal powder or the pel-

---

obscuration of the crystalline lens, the paralysis of the optic nerve, the destruction of the sense of hearing; pains also of innumerable kinds in consequence torture the patient, his mental organs suffer, his mind becomes obscured, spasmodic asthma threatens to suffocate him, or an apoplectic stroke carries him off, or some other dangerous or unbearable disease takes the place of the former ailment. Therefore the homœopathic remedy given internally must never be rubbed in on parts which suffer from external ailments.

let or pellets of the medicine have been placed. This vial is stoppered and shaken until the medicine is dissolved. From this solution one, two, three or several drops, according to the irritability and the vital force of the patient, are dropped into a cup, containing a spoonful of water; this is then well stirred and given to the patient, and where more especial care is necessary, only the half of it may be given; half a spoonful of this mixture may also well be used for the abovementioned external rubbing.

On days, when only the latter is administered, as also when it is taken internally, the little vial containing the drops must every time be briskly shaken five or six times; so also the drop or drops of medicine with the tablespoonful of water must be well stirred in the cup.

It would be still better if instead of the cup a vial should be used, into which a tablespoonful of water is put, which can then be shaken five or six times and then wholly or half emptied for a dose.

Frequently it is useful in treating chronic diseases to take the medicine, or to rub it in in the evening, shortly before going to sleep, because we have then less disturbance to fear from without, than when it is done earlier.

When I was still giving the medicines in undivided portions, each with some water at a time, I often found that the potentizing in the attenuating glasses effected by ten shakes was too strong (*i. e.*, the medicinal action too strongly developed) and I, therefore, advised only two succussions. But during the last years, since I have been giving every dose of medicine in an incorruptible solution, divided over fifteen, twenty or thirty days and even more, no potentizing in an attenuating vial is found too strong, and I again use ten strokes with each. So I herewith take back what I wrote on this subject three years ago in the first volume of this book on page 254.

In cases where a great irritability of the patient is combined with extreme debility, and the medicine can only be administered by allowing the patient to smell a few small pellets contained in a vial, when the medicine is to be used for several days, I allow the patient to smell daily of a different vial, containing the same medicine, indeed, but eyery time of a lower potency, once or twice with each nostril according as I wish him to be affected more or less.